Praise for  *'list*

"Fern Reiss has d⊙ ; together this checklist for patients u⊓... ancer treatment. Her book is well-organized and comprehensive, and fills a void in the literature. Reiss has thought of everything in this volume. As a breast surgeon, I shall recommend this book to all my patients."

—Diane Radford, M.D., FACS, FRCSEd
Breast Surgical Oncologist
Mercy Clinic St. Louis Cancer & Breast Institute

"It is a rare blessing when an oncologist gets to see something so positive come out of a patient's brush with cancer. *The Breast Cancer Checklist* is very comprehensive in its scope, clear, and incredibly helpful. This will be a wonderful guide for patients, and a very helpful teaching tool for oncology nurses, breast cancer care coordinators, and oncologists."

—Nathan Cherny, M.D.
Director, Cancer Pain and Palliative Medicine Service
Department of Medical Oncology, Shaare Zedek Medical Center

"Filled with information and advice from a survivor. I will be telling all my patients to read this book."

—Gary M. Freedman, M.D.
Associate Professor of Radiation Oncology
Perelman School of Medicine, University of Pennsylvania

The Breast Cancer Checklist
The essential guide & caring gift

The only guide with easy-to-use checklists for what to do before, during, and after breast cancer surgery, chemotherapy, and radiation, for your health, your family, and yourself. Includes:

- Checklists for pre- and post-surgery—lumpectomy, mastectomy, and reconstruction, including choosing your medical team, often overlooked medical issues, complementary medicine, managing drainage tubes, pain management, and triple-negative treatment

- Checklists for chemotherapy and radiation, infusion ports, lymphedema management, and prostheses

- Checklists for common medications including Tamoxifen, Lupron, aromatase inhibitors, and Herceptin

- Checklists for organizing your medical and insurance records, schedules, and help from family and friends

- Checklists for managing work life during treatment

- Checklists for organizing your menu planning, your treatment equipment, and clothing purchases

- Checklists of free gifts, free housecleaning, free restaurant meals, and free spa retreats & vacations

Breast cancer is stressful enough. **The Breast Cancer Checklist** will help you through it.

Other Books by Fern Reiss

The Publishing Game: Internet Publicity in 30 Days

The Publishing Game: Blog Tours in 30 Days

The Publishing Game: Bestseller in 30 Days

The Publishing Game: Publish a Book in 30 Days

The Publishing Game: Find an Agent in 30 Days

Terrorism and Kids: Comforting Your Child

The Infertility Diet: Get Pregnant and
Prevent Miscarriage

The
Breast Cancer
Checklist

by Fern Reiss

PublishingGame.com
Boston, Massachusetts

The information in this book is not intended as medical advice and should not be relied upon as a substitute for talking with your doctor and medical team. This information does not address all possible actions, precautions, interactions, and side-effects. Matters regarding your health require the supervision of a medical doctor who is familiar with your personal medical needs.

PublishingGame.com
Peanut Butter and Jelly Press, LLC
P.O. Box 590239
Newton, Massachusetts 02459-0002
(617) 630-0945
info@PBJPress.com
www.PublishingGame.com
SAN 299-7444

Library of Congress Cataloging-in-Publication Data

Reiss, Fern.
The breast cancer checklist / by Fern Reiss.
    p. cm.
Includes bibliographical references and index.
ISBN 978-1-893290-20-4
1. Breast--Cancer--Popular works. 2. Breast--Cancer--Surgery--Popular works. I. Title.
RC280.B8R45 2013
616.99'449059--dc23
                        2012027803

10 9 8 7 6 5 4 3 2 1

Dedication

To all who have gone, or are going, through the breast cancer experience, whether personally, or accompanying a friend or family member.

Thank you to my amazing international medical team: Professor Nathan Cherny, Dr. Oded Olsha, Dr. Marc Wygoda, Dr. Selwyn Strano, Dr. Chaya Rabnett, Esther Bergman, Chops Levy, Anna Kochin, Eti Yonati, Susan Ben-Dahan, Ginat and Sheldon Rice, Esther Frumkin, Ziv Rei-Korn, Rochie Schitskovsky Ivker, Rivka Nikho, and the entire nursing and support staff of Shaare Zedek Hospital in Jerusalem; Dr. Linda Vahdat; Dr. Judy Garber, Dr. Lisa Lehmann, Dr. Erin Looney, Kaitlin Sitchenko, Holly O'Kane, and the entire nursing and support staff of the Dana Farber Cancer Institute in Boston; and Dr. Judy Stone for her insight into clinical trials. Shaare Zedek, Hadassah Ein Kerem, and Dana Farber are all extraordinary medical institutions, and I'm deeply grateful to have received my care there.

And to my family, especially Jonathan, Benjamin, Daniel, and Ariel, and to my friends, for all your love and support. I couldn't have undergone this experience without you, certainly not with the clarity and confidence you provided. I'm sorry you had to share in this, but thanks so much for being there for me.

Acknowledgements

In memory of Claire Liebowitz,
from the Wiesen / Liebowitz Family

The Elster Family

In support of breast cancer warriors,
from Rabbi Bob Carroll and Ruthie Levi

Beatrice and Prof. Danny Brom

In honor of Elizabeth Tener,
from Lisa Tener

In memory of Susan Reiss Shapiro

Contents

Introduction

ော် ာ

When I was diagnosed with breast cancer two years ago, almost my first response was to head to the store to find the perfect book to get me through. But I couldn't find the book I needed.

Although I found literally hundreds of books on cancer, including dozens on breast cancer, the book I wanted wasn't there. I wasn't looking for a 500-page tome on all the intricacies and details and possibilities, though there are many excellent books on the market that provide an exhaustive (and exhausting!) look at the subject. Nor did I want narrow books specific to particular aspects of coping with breast cancer, though some of those books on lymphedema and hormone treatment are excellent.

Instead, I wanted a book that would somehow, despite the scary overtones of a cancer diagnosis, give me a feeling of control, and the ability to structure a high quality of life during my year of dealing with cancer.

I wanted a book that was quick to read, with checklists so that I wouldn't lose track of things.

I wanted an all-in-one book that I could bring with me to doctor's appointments, to the grocery store, to physical therapy, to the chemotherapy ward.

I wanted a book that didn't address just my physical condition, but also my mental and emotional condition. I wanted a book that assumed I was a cancer *survivor*, not a cancer *victim*, and one that didn't include the doom-and-gloom scenarios of cancer recurrence, which I wanted to avoid considering. I wanted a book that spoke not just to me, but also to my family, and to my friends and community, so they would know how to support me.

I even hoped for a book that would keep track of all my personal information—medical details, kids' schedules, shopping lists—so that I could stay organized and feel empowered.

This is that book. I wrote it because I needed it. I hope you find it as useful as I have.

The Top 30 Checklist

✂ ✃

If you've recently been diagnosed and you have no time to wade through this entire book... If your friend or relative is facing breast cancer treatment and you want helpful nuggets to share with them... If you just want to make sure you know the most important things... This **Top 30 Checklist** is for you.

✓	The Top 30 Checklist
	Medical
☐	**Make a dental appointment.** During treatment, you won't want to run the risk of infection, so get your teeth cleaned and any cavities filled now. (p. 57)
☐	**Get vaccinated.** See your primary care physician and get any vaccines taken care of. In particular, ask your doctor whether it's advisable for you to get a flu vaccine, a Pneumovax (pneumococcal), TDap (to protect against whooping cough), or a shingles vaccine, since your immune system will be compromised once you start chemotherapy. (p. 57)

☐	Talk to your surgeon about **cryo-preserving** your tumor, so that, should you ever need it for a personalized cancer vaccine, you have that option. (p. 58)
☐	**Ask your surgeon** if you can have your chemotherapy infusion port inserted at the same time as your breast surgery, to save you from another operation. (p. 59)

Preventative

☐	If possible, **schedule your surgery** for the second half of your menstrual cycle (i.e., days 14-29, just before you start menstruating) which seems to improve outcomes. (p. 57)
☐	A good guided **visualization tape** may lessen the pain of surgery. Make or buy a guided visualization tape so that you can better manage your pain during and after surgery. (p. 139)
☐	Be sure to **sit down with your child's teachers** and guidance counselor and make them aware of the situation, so that they're alert for mood swings and are understanding of homework snafus and absences. (p. 117)
☐	On plane flights, **wear a compression sleeve** to help

☐	prevent lymphedema. (p. 270)
	## Acquisitive
☐	**Invest in drainage tube camisoles** so that you can more easily manage (and hide) your drainage tubes after surgery. (p. 103)
☐	**Get a wig or scarf** that you'll enjoy, so that when you lose your hair, you'll have an attractive alternative to baldness. (p. 108)
☐	**Comfy cap:** Without hair, your head gets much colder, so consider a comfortable Polar Fleece cap to sleep in. Try to get one that doesn't have seams, which may irritate your scalp. (p. 108)
☐	**Try a netted bath loofah** (instead of a heavier prosthesis) for swimming: they're very lightweight and they dry quickly. (p. 203)
	## Culinary
☐	Focusing on **whole grains and vegetables,** pull together the menus that sound the best so that family members and friends can grocery shop and cook what you actually want to eat. (p. 82)
☐	**Avoid grapefruit and echinacea,** both of which can

	impede the effects of chemotherapy. (p. 214)
☐	During chemotherapy, **don't drink beverages with meals.** This simple step can forestall nausea. (p. 218)
☐	If you're taking Tamoxifen, **avoid soy:** According to the American Cancer Society, the genistein in soy can stop Tamoxifen's ability to halt breast cancer growth. (p. 244)
	## Organizational
☐	Sit down and **plan your schedule** for post-surgery and treatment, so that you fit in time for partners, kids, and yourself. (p. 131)
☐	Type up (and photocopy) a one-page **summary of all your family's needs** ('The kids have soccer practice on Tuesdays') and preferences ('Everyone loves lasagna and pizza, and I'm avoiding all sugars') so that friends can easily pitch in and help. (p. 124)
☐	Sign up for a **meal-organizing system** like CaringBridge.org or LotsaHelpingHands.com so that your friends and community can help in providing your food needs. (p. 124)
☐	**Reorganize your kitchen** (and if necessary, bathroom) so that you can easily reach everything

	you need; you'll find overhead reaching, lifting, and bending down quite challenging post-surgery. (p. 164)
☐	Investigate whether you're entitled to 12 weeks of unpaid **medical leave** from work without losing your benefits or position. (p. 153)
☐	Pre-surgery, schedule a **field trip to the hospital** with your children so that they can see where you'll be for your surgery, and for chemotherapy. Kids will feel more comfortable if they can imagine you there. Focus on the 'fun' parts of the hospital—the vending machines, the lounges, the elevators, the cafeteria, the gift shop. (p. 117)
	## Mental
☐	**Try not to let your cancer define you as a person**, and try not to let the experience of cancer completely overwhelm your year. Yes, treatment will take much of your time. But be sure you make time for other things in life, too. (p. 31)
☐	**Don't waste time obsessing** about survival rates. Survival rates have little to do with you. They're helpful for the medical establishment in understanding statistics about whole populations— but they're not talking about any particular person.

	So stay positive. (p. 30)
☐	Use your cancer experience as a way to **model behavior for your children.** At some point in their lives, they'll likely have to undergo medical treatment (or experience some other life lesson, like financial hardship); this is your opportunity to model how to behave when life hands you lemons. (p. 31)
☐	Learn how to follow-up medically **post-treatment** (p. 280) and track your follow-up care. (p. 341)
	## Hopeful
☐	**Sign up for a 'Chemo Angel'** who will send you cards and gifts to encourage you through treatment. (p. 146)
☐	**Sign up for free housecleaning** (once per month for four months) from maid services across the U.S. (p. 146)
☐	There are almost two dozen inns, spas, and retreat centers that offer free vacations to cancer survivors. **Sign up for your post-treatment vacation** now, so you can enjoy the anticipation. (p. 155)
☐	**Throw an annual "cancer-versary"** party to celebrate your cancer-free status. (p. 284)

Two Weeks Till Surgery Checklists

 os so

Most women have at least two weeks (sometimes as many as four or more) between their diagnosis and their surgery date. If you're dreading surgery, that won't seem like a short time, but there are a lot of things you'll need to get done in these few weeks.

The following chapters contain a two-week plan for you to organize your time and tasks, so that you can get everything accomplished. If it turns out that you have more time, then you can relax and move through these steps a little more slowly. In the next two weeks you will:

- Learn the basics of breast cancer—and what you'll need to do in the upcoming weeks and months ahead.

- Choose your doctors, and make your treatment decisions.

- Organize your medical records and questions for your doctors.

- Learn how to eat for breast cancer, and arrange for nutritional support.

- Organize and purchase all your needed items for surgery and beyond, including open button shirts, camisoles, and electric razors.

- Consider how to talk to friends and family about your breast cancer.

- Organize (and distribute) a family schedule to keep your family's life on track despite your treatment. Figure out when help will be needed, and arrange for carpools and the like.

- Make a guided imagery tape to improve your surgical experience. A good guided visualization tape can lessen the pain of surgery and chemotherapy.

- Learn about free opportunities including free exercise programs, restaurant meals, housecleaning, and gifts.

- Find out details about working through treatment.

- Plan your end-of-treatment (free) vacation.

- Prepare (and pack) for your hospital stay.

- Take a mini-vacation.

The rest of the book contains detailed checklists for guiding you through post-surgery recovery, drainage care, pain management, infusion port insertion, prosthesis purchase, chemotherapy, radiation, Herceptin, Tamoxifen, Lupron, aromatase inhibitors, triple-negative diagnoses, lymphedema management, clinical trials, post-treatment, and more.

Day 1:
Think About the Basics

CB BO

Everyone is different, and everyone's breast cancer is different. So while this book aims to be a checklist that every breast cancer patient can use to navigate through the journey, you may find parts of it useful and parts of it less useful. Use what works for you, and ignore the rest. Here are some good ideas to start with:

- Don't gulp. Take it one step at a time, slowly. Although your medical team, post-diagnosis, will want to start treatment, another few days will not affect your prognosis. Take the time to get a second opinion, to read the research, to ask questions, and to organize your treatment plan. Don't let yourself be panicked into rushing.

- Take the time to look carefully through this book and notice the sections where you can track your information. If you keep your receipts and records and details all together, it will make you less frenetic when you need to locate a particular fact or item; being organized will simplify your experience.

- Don't spend a lot of your time worrying about survival rates. Survival rates really don't have anything to do with *you*. They're helpful for the medical establishment in understanding statistics about whole populations—but they're not talking about any particular person. Your survival is as good as you think it will be—so stay positive, make some healthy lifestyle changes, and be certain you're going to survive. That's the single best thing you can do for your survival.

- Try not to feed into your stress. Getting a cancer diagnosis isn't fun for anyone. Take it in and try to do your best to move on. Your condition isn't going to improve if you obsess about it. Imagine yourself treating your condition calmly and clearly.

- Nor will you help yourself by taking in your disease passively. Visualize yourself being in control of your disease and your treatment. Take charge of whatever sounds reasonable to you without being overwhelming: your diet, your exercise plan, your treatment. Just the empowering feeling of being in control, with an active role, will help tremendously in the mind-body component of your cancer. Keep in mind that studies have hinted that there's a correlation between belief that your treatment plan will work, and effectiveness/cure rates. So hunt down the best treatment plan you can—and then believe in it wholeheartedly.

- Try not to let cancer define you as a person, and try not to let the experience of cancer completely overwhelm your year. Yes, you have cancer; yes, treating that cancer will take a lot of your time and energy this year. But be sure you make time for other things in life too.

- See your cancer diagnosis as a challenge, and an opportunity, rather than a sentence. View it as a way to reprioritize your life, and a way to take back your time, and reallocate it in a more effective and more aligned-with-your-values way. Regard it as an opportunity to repair relationships that have strayed, and to form new friendships and family ties.

- Use your cancer experience as a way to model behavior for your children: At some point, they'll also have to undergo some sort of medical treatment (or experience some other life lesson, like financial hardship or personal loss); this is your opportunity to model for them how to behave when life hands you lemons.

- Use your cancer diagnosis to change your life. If not now, when?

- And make sure you're enjoying your life. Yes, even during this year of breast cancer. Delight in the little things: A food that you don't usually eat. A walk through the park. A coffee date with a friend. A snuggle with your child. Pay attention to the small things that give you pleasure, and vow to do more of them. As much as possible, live for the moment. Make sure you're taking time to play and laugh.

Day 2:
Make Some Medical Decisions

C06 80

Most doctors will want to schedule you for surgery as quickly as their calendars will allow; you will likely have just a few weeks between diagnosis and surgery. Not everyone will need chemotherapy, but if you do, then the doctor will likely want to start the chemotherapy within a month of your surgery date (unless your oncologist decides on pre-surgery chemotherapy).

Treatment Options

Depending on the type and extent of your breast cancer, the medical team will usually recommend one of the three following protocols:

- Lumpectomy (to remove just the breast lump) followed by chemotherapy (sometimes) and radiation therapy (almost always).

- Mastectomy (to remove the entire breast or both breasts) followed by chemotherapy (usually) and radiation therapy (if any lymph nodes were affected)

- Chemotherapy (also called neoadjuvant therapy) to shrink a particularly large or aggressive tumor, followed by surgery (either lumpectomy or mastectomy), and then often radiation therapy (if radiation was not given pre-surgery)

Chemotherapy means treatment with cancer-killing drugs.

Radiation therapy means treatment with a beam of high-energy x-rays, otherwise known as *external beam radiation*, for six to eight weeks; or (sometimes) internal radiation therapy, also known as *brachytherapy*, where a radioactive material is inserted into the lumpectomy site, typically for a few minutes at a time, twice a day, for five days.

In addition, as part of the surgery, doctors may recommend either:

- Lymph node removal, also known as axillary lymph node dissection, where the surgeon removes 10 to 40 lymph nodes to evaluate for cancer spread, or

- Sentinel node biopsy, in which the surgeon injects dye into the breast to find, remove, and then check just the first ("sentinel") lymph nodes into which the tumor drains, as they're the most likely to contain cancerous cells; if they are cancer-free, there is no need to remove further lymph nodes.

Details of reconstruction are explored in the chapter on reconstruction (p. 69), but you'll need to decide whether to:

- Forego reconstruction (and perhaps use a prosthesis/breast form)

- Have immediate reconstruction (in which case, if you're scheduled for a mastectomy, your surgeon may recommend a skin-sparing mastectomy or nipple-sparing mastectomy, where most of the skin over the breast and/or the nipple is left intact, which results in less scarring)

- Have delayed reconstruction (to allow your body to recover from the effects of the first surgery)

You'll want to consider whether you should participate in a clinical trial for chemotherapy or supportive care. Clinical trials are not only last-resort options; there are many clinical trials that look at trying to improve quality-of-life during and after treatment. You might also benefit by receiving the newest treatment and having additional care and attention from the clinical trial staff. More information can be found in the clinical trials chapter, p. 277.

You'll want to select a medical team and doctors who:

- Are easy to speak with (and make themselves available)

- Have good reputations and references

- Are optimistic and encouraging about your prognosis

Unfortunately, it's probably not going to be as easy as going to one doctor and stopping there. There will probably be multiple doctors involved in your treatment; they may not always agree with each other; and depending on your feelings about complementary medicine and how much complementary medicine you want to incorporate into your treatment plan, they may not even all speak with each other.

At times it may feel easier to just throw up your hands and choose one specialist. But your health may be compromised if you don't spend some time and energy incorporating various medical viewpoints, and reading the literature yourself. Ultimately, it's your health—and your decision.

Checklist: Making Appointments

Once you have evaluated your treatment options, it's time to make appointments to choose a doctor. Here are some things to consider:

✓	Making Appointments
☐	See a specialist. Don't get an opinion on breast cancer from a general surgeon; see an oncological surgeon.
☐	Get two opinions. Doctors do not always agree, either on diagnosis (what you have) or prognosis (likely outcome based on your treatment plan) so it's important to hear from more than one doctor so you really know what your options are. (Second opinions are standard procedure, so doctors won't be offended.) The cost of a second opinion is almost always reimbursed in full by medical insurance.
☐	See a specialist in a different practice for your second opinion. Choose doctors in two different cancer treatment centers so they have no connection with each other—and no vested reason to agree with the opinion you've already gotten.
☐	Be sure that you're consulting with doctors that work with a team; ideally, a surgeon, medical oncologist, and radiation oncologist should all be

	involved in your diagnosis and treatment plan, because they'll all be viewing your cancer through the lens of their specialty (surgery, chemotherapy, radiation), and you'll want to hear all those views before you make treatment decisions. You may be told that you'll need all three treatment protocols, but it's still best to ask specialists in different areas so you really know what your options are.
☐	While you're at the hospital, schedule an appointment with the social worker. Some hospitals have social workers who work specifically in the oncology ward. The hospital social worker will be able to tell you about all of the programs and benefits available to cancer patients.
☐	Remember to bring all your medical records and test results to all appointments with doctors so that you're operating from a place of similar information. Doctors will want to see actual pathology slides, not just reports, plus film/images on disc.
☐	Bring a tape-recorder to all doctor's appointments, and record your discussions. It can be difficult to assimilate information (and remember it) amidst the emotion of diagnosis and treatment, and having a recording of your discussion can be extremely helpful later on.
☐	Ask a spouse or friend to accompany you to all doctor's appointments. Most people find it difficult

	to be their own advocate in the medical system, and it's very helpful to have someone else along to assimilate information, ask questions, and later recall what was discussed.
☐	Create a folder in which to house all receipts and medical correspondence. That way, even if it takes you time to sort through the folder each time you need a receipt or paper, at least you know that everything you need is in there.

Fill-in: Recommended Doctors

Recommended Doctors		
Doctor / Practice	Recommended By	Comments

Doctor / Practice	Recommended By	Comments

Checklist: Doctor Preview

✓	Doctor Preview
☐	Ask friends for recommendations of doctors
☐	Make a list of the doctors
☐	Narrow down your list to two or three doctors
☐	Call the doctor's offices and explain your situation to the nurse or receptionist
☐	Ask with which hospital or cancer center the doctor is affiliated
☐	Schedule an appointment to meet the doctor
☐	Ask the nurse if it's better to bring or send your medical records
☐	Verify that the doctor accepts your insurance
☐	Call your insurance company to verify that this doctor is covered by your policy
☐	Confirm that insurance will cover a second opinion
☐	Gather your medical records and diagnostic reports to bring (or send) to the doctor's visit
☐	Bring any x-rays, mammograms, MRIs, PET and CT

	scans to your appointment
☐	Bring *Your Medical Profile* (p. 42) to all appointments, even if you've already mailed your information

Other things you may want to do before your appointment:

- Fill out your family health history with the free online tool at *familyhistory.hhs.gov*.

- Check out the list of current recommendations for treating your type of breast cancer at the National Comprehensive Cancer Network (*www.nccn.org*).

Fill-in: Your Medical Profile

Save time by compiling the following medical details and information which your doctors will need. Your doctors will keep your official medical charts, but keep your own records, so that when other doctors, nurses, and medical care providers ask you questions, you have the answers at your fingertips. You might want to photocopy these pages (bringing a copy to each doctor's appointment) so that doctors can easily attach the info to their records.

Your Medical Profile	
Date of birth	
Height and weight	
Insurance plan and membership number	
Date of last menstrual period	
At what age did your periods begin? (At what age did they end, if post-menopausal?)	
When was your last tetanus shot?	
Have you had a flu or pneumonia vaccine this year?	
Have you ever had surgery?	
Do you have any medical conditions?	

Do you smoke/drink/use drugs?	
Have you ever had cancer? Where?	
Do your mother or sisters have a history of breast cancer? Ovarian cancer?	
Do your father or brothers have a history of prostate cancer? (Breast, ovarian, and prostate cancer share a genetic component.)	
Does anyone else in your family have a history of breast, ovarian, or prostate cancer? Any other cancer?	

Do you (or do any family members) test positive for the BRCA gene mutations?	
What food supplements and vitamins do you take?	
Do you have allergies or reactions to medications?	
What medications do you take?	

Fill-in: Choosing a Doctor

Here are questions to ask when deciding on a doctor (ask if you can tape record your conversation; that way, you'll have an accurate record when you get home):

Choosing a Doctor	
Doctor's name	
Name of practice	
Secretary / receptionist	
Address	
Phone/fax	
E-mail address	
Does your practice accept my insurance?	
Are there any fees my health insurance won't cover of which I should be aware?	
At which hospital(s) do you have	

privileges?	
Where will I do my surgery?	
With which oncologists, surgeons, and radiation oncologists do you work?	
With which plastic surgeons do you work?	
Where will I do my chemotherapy?	
Where will I do my radiation therapy?	
If you're recommending a lumpectomy, can we discuss brachytherapy instead of traditional (external beam) radiation? And if so, can I have the balloon catheter	

inserted at the same time as my lumpectomy? (See p. 59)	
How long have you been in practice?	
Which medical school did you attend?	
How many of these surgeries do you do per month / year?	
Will I have appointments with anyone else in your practice?	
How far in advance do I need to schedule appointments?	
How often will I have appointments?	
What days of the week can I schedule	

appointments?	
What are hours on weekends?	
Can I call or email the office with questions? How soon will I be called back?	
What type of breast cancer do I have?	
What stage of breast cancer do I have?	
What grade of breast cancer do I have?	
Can you explain my pathology report?	
What did the mammogram or biopsy reveal?	
Has the cancer spread to lymph nodes or other organs?	

Do I have estrogen- or progesterone-positive tumors, and what does that mean in terms of treatment?	
Do I have HER2/neu-positive tumors, and what does that mean in terms of treatment?	
Should I get a 2nd opinion on the tissue samples?	
What are my options for treatment?	
What treatment is most appropriate for me? Why?	
What are the short and long-term side-effects of the treatment?	
Can we do anything to prevent the side-	

effects?	
Will I go through menopause as a result of my treatment?	
Will I be able to have children after my treatment?	
When is the earliest date for which I can schedule surgery?	
Are you in town the weeks just before and after my scheduled surgery?	
What post-operative symptoms should I be sure to call about? (Anything I should go to the hospital for?)	
What kind of post-surgery pain options will I have?	

Can you tell me how long I will have to have drains in, and how I manage those? (See p. 181)	
Can I use a guided visualization tape during my surgery? (i.e., Is it ok with you if I use head-phones)? (See p. 139)	
Can I cryo-preserve my tumor? (See p. 58)	
Post-surgery, when can I engage in normal activities? Exercising? Driving? Working? Sex?	
Do you recommend that I get an infusion port? Can I get that inserted at the same time as my surgery? (See p. 197)	

Should I get genetic testing?	
Should I look into clinical trials? (See p. 277)	
Tell me about reconstruction. If I want it, should I do it now or later? (See p. 69)	
What do I need to do to prepare for surgery and treatment? (See p. 163)	
Might I need a blood transfusion, and should I bank my own blood?	
Should I get a flu vaccine, Pneumovax, Tdap, or a shingles vaccine now (before chemotherapy)?	
Should I make	

lifestyle changes? Nutritional changes?	
What are my odds of recurrence with the treatment you've outlined? What happens then?	
What will be the effects of this treatment on my day-to-day life? What changes should I expect to make? What will my energy level be? Can I / should I exercise? Will I be able to work during treatment? Travel?	
How successful is this treatment protocol for the type of cancer I have?	
How will you ascertain whether/how well	

it's working?	
What is the timetable for treatments? How long do I need to wait between treatments? How long will the total treatment regimen take?	
What should my next steps be?	
What medications, vitamins, and supplements should I stop taking before the surgery, and how far in advance should I stop?	
Are there any special vitamins or supplements I should start?	
Tell me about birth control during	

treatment.	
Do I have a choice between outpatient or in-patient surgery?	
How long will my surgery take?	
Can I schedule the surgery for my luteal phase? (See p. 57)	
Is there a social worker associated with the hospital whom I can see? (Get name, contact details, and hours available, and make an appointment.)	
If I'm scheduled for a full axillary lymph node dissection, can I have a referral to an occupational or physical therapist for baseline arm measurements pre-	

surgery (for later lymphedema issues)? (See p. 267)	
Is there anything I've forgotten to ask?	

Checklist: Overlooked Medical Issues

These are the details most often overlooked by women in breast cancer treatment, so add them to your list!

✓	Overlooked Medical Issues
☐	**Get dental work.** During chemotherapy you'll be at increased risk of infection, so make a dental appointment and get any cleanings and fillings that you'll need out of the way.
☐	**Get vaccinated.** Similarly, since you'll be immuno-compromised during chemotherapy and won't want to be vaccinated, ask your doctor about getting any necessary vaccines now, including a flu vaccine, Pneumovax, Tdap, and a shingles vaccine.
☐	**Time your surgery** for the second half of your cycle. If you are given a choice, keep in mind that there is some evidence, based on medical studies, that you'll improve your outcome if you time your surgery based on your menstrual cycle. Pre-menopausal

	women who schedule their mastectomy during the luteal (second) phase of their menstrual cycle seem to have a lower recurrence risk. So, for example, if the first day of your menstrual cycle (i.e., the first day of bleeding) is day number one, schedule your surgery for days 14-29 (that is, right before you start menstruating again), rather than earlier. If you don't have control over your surgery date because of the surgeon's or hospital's schedule, or you're in perimenopause and can't predict your menstrual cycle, don't fret: The evidence on this is by no means conclusive, and few surgeons inquire about menstrual cycles as a way of setting surgery dates.
☐	**Cryo-preserve** your tumor. You may feel like a character in a Woody Allen movie, but consider cryo-preserving your tumor. One of the most promising advances is an in-development cancer vaccine which works by reintroducing the body's own tumor (along with something that the body recognizes as harmful) so that the body learns to fight the tumor cells. By cryo-preserving your original tumor, you'll have tumor cells should you ever need them for a tailored vaccine. There are cryo-preservation facilities across the country and the cost is not exorbitant. Most doctors won't be familiar with this request, but will probably be able to accommodate you.
☐	**Check on egg freezing.** If you plan to someday have

(more) children, ask your doctor about freezing your embryos or eggs before undergoing treatment. Cancer treatment, particularly chemotherapy, can push you (possibly prematurely) into menopause, so since you may stop ovulating as a result, consider taking fertility drugs and freezing your eggs before you start treatment if this is a consideration. An egg-retrieval cycle typically takes 2-4 weeks.

Women concerned about their fertility should be in touch with Fertile Hope, *FertileHope.org*, (888) 994-2353, or the Oncofertility Consortium (*oncofertility. northwestern.edu*) hotline, (866) 708-3378. *MyOncoFertility.org* is another resource for patients provided by the Oncofertility Consortium.

☐ **Schedule simultaneous surgeries.** Before you schedule surgery, ask your surgeon if it's possible to have the reconstructive surgery at the same time as your surgery. (Depending on the complexity of your situation, this may be a possibility.)

☐ **Schedule simultaneous port insertion.** If you're going to need chemotherapy, ask your surgeon whether the infusion port can be implanted at the same time as your surgery. Otherwise, this will require an additional surgical procedure.

☐ **Schedule simultaneous brachytherapy catheter implantation.** If you're having a lumpectomy and are a candidate for brachytherapy (internal radiation

	therapy) rather than traditional (external beam radiation) therapy, ask your surgeon whether the balloon catheter can be implanted at the same time as your lumpectomy. Otherwise, you will require an additional surgical procedure.

Checklist: Get Organized for Insurance

✓	Get Organized for Insurance
☐	Look through your insurance policy to verify what is covered
☐	Call your insurance company and have someone walk you through what's covered, what needs a co-pay, and what other services (e.g. physical therapy, lymphedema treatment) are included in your policy.
☐	Fill out the insurance summary on p. 299 so you can easily answer questions about co-pays and deductibles.
☐	Get into the habit of immediately photocopying any surgical records, new lab test results, or follow-ups to put into your folder, so you always have extra copies to hand out at doctor appointments.
☐	Track treatment details on the forms in the appendices: • Treatment Summary, p. 315

	• Surgeries, p. 321 • Diagnostic tests, p. 325 • Doctor appointments, p. 333 • Medications, p. 339
☐	Be sure you've set up a system to pay insurance premiums on time to keep your coverage active. If your policy lapses, it will be difficult to find new coverage at low cost because you now have a "pre-existing condition".
☐	Be sure you're following the insurance plan's 'rules' for treatment approval (e.g. get a second opinion, make sure your primary care physician is making the referral, etc.)
☐	Keep track of all interactions with the insurance company (see p. 301)
☐	Ask your insurance company if there's a designated mail-order company for drug purchases, which can potentially save a lot of money. Track these purchases carefully (see p. 309).
☐	Keep track of mileage and/or expenses associated with each trip to doctors, hospitals, diagnostic tests, physical therapy appointments, pharmacies, etc., all of which might be able to be written off your taxes (see p. 307).

☐	Keep careful records of all medical treatment and insurance plan payments (see p. 305).

Complementary Treatment

There is a growing body of evidence that using the mind/body connection can help in your recovery. Since lifestyle choices such as attitude, self-care, nutrition, exercise, family and community support, and spirituality can be contributing factors to your medical condition, improving those choices may, along with traditional medical treatment, be efficacious in improving your condition.

Contrastingly, alternatives that are not safe and not efficacious can delay or impede treatment, and should be avoided.

As soon as your diagnosis is public, people will come out of the woodwork to tell you about alternative ways to treat your cancer. These methods may include vitamins, herbs and special diets, or other methods such as acupuncture and massage, to name just a few.

Although faced with the difficult regimen of surgery and chemotherapy it can be tempting to opt for side-effect-free massage instead, keep in mind that many alternative treatments, while good **additions** to traditional treatment, are not good **substitutes** for traditional treatment.

So in addition to undergoing conventional medical care (surgery, chemotherapy, radiation, etc.), consider integrating complementary approaches into your treatment. There is mounting medical evidence that including certain complementary approaches in a conventional treatment plan will yield better results, as well as reduced side-effects and higher quality of life, and a growing number of traditional doctors are willing to work with their patients to integrate holistic therapies.

Moreover, incorporating holistic approaches in your treatment plan is likely to reduce stress effectively, might improve pain management, and can give you a greater sense of control over your disease.

If one of the following resonates for you, consider adding it as an adjunct to your treatment:

- Meditation, biofeedback, guided imagery, yoga, expressive arts (music, art, or dance) therapy
- Macrobiotic or vegan diet, herbal remedies, vitamins, dietary supplements
- Massage, reflexology
- Reiki, therapeutic touch, magnetic field therapy
- Traditional Chinese medicine, including acupuncture, ayurvedic medicine, homeopathy, naturopathic medicine

Fill-in:
Complementary Treatment Appointments

Questions to ask in looking for complementary treatment:

Complementary Treatment Appointments	
Name of doctor / therapist	
Name of practice	
Address	
Phone / fax	
E-mail	
Cost	
Does your practice accept my insurance?	
How long have you been in practice?	
What can I expect to get out of this treatment?	

Is this treatment specifically recommended for breast cancer?	
How often is recommended treatment? For how many weeks?	
Do I need to bring or wear anything special?	
Directions	
Is there anything else I've forgotten to ask?	

Fill-in: Complementary Treatment Classes

Questions to ask in looking for complementary classes:

Complementary Treatment Classes	
Class	
Address	
Phone/fax	
Email	
Name of instructor(s)	
How much does it cost?	
Is it covered by my health insurance plan?	
How many weeks is the course?	
Are there shorter/longer versions?	

How long is each class?	
Do I need to bring anything with me (swimsuit, towel, flip-flops, yoga mat) or wear any particular kind of clothing (loose-fitting clothes, easy-to-slip-off shoes, etc)?	
How many people are in each class?	
When does the session start? End?	
How much does it cost?	
Directions	

Day 3: Reconstruction

∞ ∞

The decision about whether to have reconstructive surgery after lumpectomy or mastectomy is an individual one. You can have reconstruction at the same time as your surgery, you can have it later, or you don't have to have it at all. Even if you're planning to wait and have it later, speak to your surgeon as well as a plastic surgeon **before** your surgery to determine the treatment plan that's best for you.

Reconstruction Options

There are many methods of reconstruction, but the two most common types are:

- Tissue expander—saline breast implants, where a tissue expander that stretches the skin is surgically placed beneath the major chest muscle, saline solution is injected over a period of months, and finally, breast implants are surgically inserted (silicone implants are also possible but now less common)

- Muscle flap reconstruction, where your own tissue is removed from your back, abdomen, or buttocks to rebuild the breast, and microsurgically connected to the blood vessels in the chest region.

  o With the latissimus dorsi flap, muscle, fat, and skin from your upper back creates a pocket for an implant. Some women experience weakness in their back and shoulders afterwards.

  o With the TRAM flap, muscle, fat, and skin from your abdomen may be enough to shape the breast, without the necessity for an implant, though it can affect abdominal strength. TRAM flaps can either be pedicle flaps (where the flap is tunneled up through the chest wall remaining attached to its original blood supply) or free flaps (where the flap is cut loose of its original location and then reattached in the chest area microsurgically.)

  o With the DIEP (deep inferior epigastric artery perforator) free flap, fat tissue from your abdominal area (but **not** the muscle) forms the breast mound, resulting in a 'tummy tuck.' The procedure causes fewer hernias and less muscle weakness than the TRAM pedicle flap.

  o With the GAP free flap or SGAP flap, fat tissue (but not muscle) from the buttocks is used.

  o With the TUG free flap, fatty tissue from the bottom of the buttocks to the inner thigh is used, making it particularly appropriate for women with fat thighs.

Considerations in Reconstruction

Here are some things to consider:

- Don't be pushed into plastic surgery just because you're speaking to a plastic surgeon.

- Don't be pushed into a particular kind of reconstruction just because you're speaking to a plastic surgeon who specializes in it.

- Don't feel rushed into deciding on reconstruction prematurely. Delaying reconstruction can be a way to see if you adjust to living without your breasts. You have time to research the options and consider the alternatives.

- Be aware that reconstruction can cause infection, which may cause your chemotherapy or radiation to be delayed.

- Often, reconstructive surgery requires more than one operation.

- Immediate reconstruction (done by a plastic surgeon right after the general surgeon does the lumpectomy or mastectomy) reduces the discomfort of two major operations and may reduce the expense as well. However, it's more likely to result in necrosis (cell death) or infection of the breast; if this occurs, more surgery will be needed to fix the situation. Immediate reconstruction can be a good choice for women who don't need radiation.

- Staged or delayed reconstruction involves several surgeries over at least six months. Delayed reconstruction is a better choice for women who will need radiation, as radiation post-reconstruction can be problematic, particularly in women receiving tissue expander-implant surgery.

- Nipple and areola reconstruction are available as a separate surgery (and the last stage of reconstruction). You can do this as an outpatient under local anesthesia, usually 3-4 months after the breast reconstruction.

- Surgeons may offer surgery to reshape the remaining breast to match the reconstructed breast. Insurance won't always automatically cover this cost, though— oncological and plastic surgeons may have to petition and make a case for this coverage.

- Flap procedures leave two scar sites—at the reconstructed breast, and also at the spot where the tissue was removed.

- Abdominal hernias and muscle damage are possibilities.

- Women who smoke or have diabetes are usually ineligible for flap procedures.

- Smokers will be advised to quit smoking for at least 2-3 weeks before reconstructive surgery to ensure proper healing (thus making delayed reconstruction their best option). Surgeons can test urine the day of surgery to ensure that smoking has really stopped.

- Flaps don't rupture.

- Reconstructed breasts won't have sensation.

- Flap surgery can result in a loss of sensation at the donor site (as well as the breast).

- Incision lines will always be visible, both at the breast and at the donor site (abdomen, back, buttocks).

- Breast implants can rupture, causing infection and/or pain. Some estimates suggest as many as half of implants may need to be replaced within ten years, requiring more surgery.

- Breast implants can end up unnaturally firm, with scar tissue hardening around the implants (capsular contracture).

- Routine mammograms on breast implants are difficult.

- Unless mastectomies were performed, breast implants post-augmentation should have no effect on breastfeeding.

- If you have TRAM or DIEP reconstruction with abdominal tissue on a unilateral mastectomy, and you later decide to have the other breast removed, you can't repeat the procedure.

- You'll recover from implant reconstruction faster than flap reconstruction, but both require at least 4-6 weeks of recovery. You'll need to refrain from strenuous activity, overhead lifting, and sexual activity during recovery.

- If you don't reconstruct you can resume normal activity earlier.   Mastectomy without reconstruction will involve less recovery time, and fewer complications.

- Bilateral reconstruction with TRAM flaps is discouraged because of permanent abdominal strength loss.

- If you don't reconstruct you won't have to have additional surgery on your back, abdomen, or buttocks, and won't risk loss of muscle function there.

- Should your cancer recur, post-implant recurrences are usually in front of the muscle and can be detected; post-flap (behind the flap) recurrences are extremely rare.

- Flap procedures involve a shorter reconstruction process, but a more difficult recovery. Tissue expander reconstruction involves an easier recovery than flap procedures, but a lengthier reconstruction process: many doctor visits and surgeries over the course of six months is usual.

- Even women who have had reconstruction may find that they need partial prostheses and mastectomy bras. See p. 201 for more details on bra solutions post-reconstruction.

Nipple and Areola Reconstruction

Finally, you'll need to decide if you want your nipple and areola (the dark area around the nipple) reconstructed.

- Nipple/areola reconstruction is a separate (optional) surgery.

- It's usually done four months after the rest of the reconstruction is complete, and under local anesthesia.

- The tissue to rebuild is taken from elsewhere in your body (usually from your groin, thigh, or buttocks.)

- The surgeon will often use a tattoo to match the color of the other nipple.

- In women with small, early-stage cancer, it's sometimes possible to do a nipple- or areola-sparing mastectomy, where the nipple and/or areola are left while the breast tissue is removed. Because of the poor blood supply, sometimes (about 10% of the time) the nipple withers or becomes misshapen, and there is rarely much feeling in the nipple.

Fill-in:
Choosing a Reconstruction Surgeon

Questions to ask when deciding on a plastic surgeon. (Ask if you can tape record your conversation, so you'll have an accurate record when you get home.)

Choosing a Reconstruction Surgeon	
Doctor's name	
Name of practice	
Secretary / receptionist	
Address	
Phone/fax	
E-mail address	
Does your practice accept my insurance?	
Are there any fees my health insurance won't cover of which I should be aware?	
At which hospital(s) do you have	

privileges?	
Can you work with the oncological surgeon I've chosen?	
Am I a candidate for breast reconstruction?	
What types of reconstruction can I have?	
What type of reconstruction is best for me? Why?	
What can I expect the result to be?	
How long have you been in practice? Where is your degree from? How many of these surgeries do you do per month / year?	
Will I have appointments with anyone else in your	

practice?	
How far in advance do I need to schedule appointments?	
How often will I need to have appointments?	
Can I call or email the office with questions? How soon will I be called back?	
What's the earliest date for which I can schedule surgery?	
Are you in town the weeks just before and after my scheduled surgery?	
Of what possible problems should I be aware?	
Will I have pain or scarring? Will I have	

changes in the parts of my body from which the tissue is being taken?	
How much pain will I suffer?	
How long will I stay in the hospital?	
How long will the recovery be?	
What will I need to do at home to care for my incision?	
When can I engage in normal activities? Exercising? Driving? Working? Sex?	
Will reconstruction interfere with my chemotherapy or radiation?	
How long are the breast implants expected to last?	

How will aging and weight changes affect the reconstructed breast?	
What medicines, vitamins, and supplements should I discontinue before surgery?	
What medicines, vitamins, and supplements should I begin taking before surgery?	
How long before surgery should I stop eating and drinking?	
How long before surgery should I discontinue aspirin and other NSAIDs?	
Is there anything I've forgotten to ask?	

Day 4:
Diet and Exercise

☞ ☜

I inadvertently gave two women quite a thrill. After eight months of my very restrictive diet, I was sitting in a coffee shop with a friend, regaling her enthusiastically with my ongoing craving for a grilled cheese sandwich "I can't stop fantasizing about it, I just can't stop thinking about it, I obsess about it all the time, I can't get any work done because I can't get my mind off it, I'm thinking about cheating all the time and I'm having all these fantasies... Do you think it would hurt if I cheated just once?" Suddenly, my friend kicked me and said "Hush!" She had noticed that the two nearby women were eavesdropping so avidly that they had almost toppled over onto our table. My friend hissed, "They think you're talking about something else!" (Seems they hadn't heard the first line of my fantasy conversation and thought we were having quite a different conversation—"I'll have what she had.")

An increasing number of women in treatment view food as medicine. So, soon after their diagnosis, they search for nutritional plans designed to aid in their recovery.

Many doctors tend to disregard nutritional adjuncts to traditional treatment, but although the medical studies examining nutritional links to breast cancer can be contradictory, eating more healthfully (and altering your diet to consume more things like broccoli) probably can't hurt and are worth a try. Here are some ideas to get you started.

Diet Suggestions

- **Eat whole grains.** Eat brown rice rather than white, whole wheat bread instead of white bread, whole grain pasta instead of white pasta, etc. Keep in mind that even whole-grain pasta is a mix of whole wheat and white, unless it's marked 100% whole wheat.[1,2,3,9,13,15]

- **Add more vegetables**[4,5,9,11,12,13] **and fruit**[4,7,8,12,13] to your diet.

- **Add more fish**[6,15,39] to your diet. Oily fish, such as salmon and sardines, are particularly rich in vitamin D, which, along with vitamin D from sun exposure, helps prevent breast cancer.[25]

- **Decrease your consumption of meat,**[9,10,11,15] **chicken, eggs, and high-fat dairy** (low-fat and fermented dairy products associate with decreased risk).[14]

- **Reduce your sugar intake.** Unfortunately, this includes everything from refined sugar, to maple syrup and honey, to any other kind of sweetener including white bread and excessive fruit.[2,15,23]

The most recent guidelines from the American Cancer Society recommend limiting intake of high-calorie foods and drinks.[16] They say:

> *Does sugar increase cancer risk? Sugar increases calorie intake without providing any of the nutrients that reduce cancer risk. By promoting obesity, a high sugar intake may indirectly increase cancer risk. White (refined) sugar is no different from brown (unrefined) sugar or honey with regard to their effects on body weight or insulin levels. Limiting foods such as cakes, candy, cookies, and sweetened cereals, as well as sugar-sweetened drinks such as soda and sports drinks can help reduce calorie intake.[17]*

o Sugar:

   ▪ Suppresses your body's immune function, and

   ▪ Causes unhealthy extreme insulin fluctuations[18]

o ER-negative, and particularly ER-negative post-menopausal women, should be careful about sugar, according to new studies linking high-glycemic index food (sugar, white carbohydrates, etc.) to a particularly deadly form of breast cancer in ER-negative women.[12,19]

- o Older women also show a higher correlation between breast cancer mortality and sugar consumption.[21]

- As much as possible, **eat less-processed** foods.

- **Drink—and drink water.** Studies seem to indicate that chronic dehydration can increase breast cancer rates significantly.[28] Sodas are diuretics that drain the body of water unnecessarily and fruit juice has too much sugar.

- **Tea** slows tumor growth[29]. Green tea seems to be particularly helpful.[30,68] **Coffee** seems to reduce the risk of breast cancer particularly in postmenopausal women with ER-negative tumors.[24]

- **Eat beans**, and other legumes including lentils, peas, and peanuts.[1]

- **Eat tomatoes.** The lycopene in tomatoes is thought to be helpful. Apricots, guava, watermelon, papaya, and pink grapefruit also have high lycopene content.[31,32]

- **Eat cruciferous vegetables**, including broccoli, cauliflower, cabbage, and collard greens. All cruciferous vegetables contain phenylethyl isothiocyanate, which seems to kill cancer cells; they also contain indole-3-carbinol, which helps block cancer metastasis.[34,35]

- **Eat raw broccoli.** Broccoli contains sulforaphane, which helps; high consumption of sulforaphane also apparently leads to lower cancer recurrence rates.[27] Cooking can break down the active ingredients, so eat it raw if possible.[36]

- **Combining certain foods** can also heighten their effectiveness (because they'll be better absorbed, or because the foods work better in concert) so for example pairing tomatoes and broccoli[37]; avocado and carrots; blueberries and apples; and spinach and strawberries will increase the tumor-fighting abilities of any of the foods eaten separately.

- **Eat kale** and other green leafy vegetables high in vitamin K.[38] **Parsley** and **celery** with their high apigenin levels also have preventative properties.[22]

- **Eat apples, red onions,** and (again) **kale** (as well as leafy green vegetables, tea, berries, and red wine) all of which contain quercetin. Promising early studies indicate that the quercetin has anti-inflammatory properties.[40,41]

- **Eat onions** and **garlic** both of which correlate with reduced cancer risk.[42,45]

- **Eat mushrooms.** The beta-glucans in mushrooms can reportedly both enhance the effectiveness of chemotherapy, while reducing side-effects. Maitake, shiitake, and reishi mushrooms are all useful.[43,44,68]

- **Eat spices.** Natural anti-inflammatory phytochemicals in spices including turmeric,[45,46] red pepper,[45] cloves,[45] cumin,[45] rosemary,[45,48] anise,[45] fennel,[45] basil,[45] and ginger[45,49] are good; they're also thought to inhibit the growth of HER2/neu cells. Also good is cardamom.[47]

- **Eat nuts**, especially walnuts, peanuts, pecans, and chestnuts for their antioxidant properties.[50] Walnuts also have anti-inflammatory properties,[33] and seem to slow cancer growth.[20] Nut consumption helps prevent cancer.[1,51]

- **Citrus fruit peel and oil** have anti-tumor properties.[52]

- **Eat seaweed** (nori, kombu, kelp, dulse, arame, wakame, and hijiki) which can help activate your body's cancer-fighting cells.[53]

- **Eat watercress.** The phenylethyl isothiocyanate in watercress can block a tumor's ability to grow new blood cells, effectively starving the tumor of essential blood and oxygen.[54]

- **Eat berries**[56] **and pomegranates.**[45,55] Phytochemicals in these foods seem to inhibit breast cancer; they're also powerful anti-inflammatories. The bromelain in **pineapple** is also an anti-inflammatory.[57]

- **Eat chocolate.** Compounds in chocolate act as antioxidants, and combat cell damage that can lead to tumor growth. (But milk chocolate with a high sugar content isn't good for you, so stick to dark chocolate, at least 80%, where sugar is not the first ingredient).[58]

- **Flax seed,**[61] **sesame seed,** cruciferous vegetables like broccoli and cabbage, and apricots and strawberries, all with their high lignan levels, might be helpful in reducing your risk for breast cancer, particularly in overweight pre-menopausal women,[59] and post-menopausal women.[60,62] Seeds of all sorts (sunflower, pumpkin, as well as flax and sesame) are effective.[1] Sesame seeds, in particular, protect against inflammation.[33]

- **Try to stick to olive oil.** Olive oil is an anti-inflammatory, and may reduce the risk of breast and other cancers.[13,15,26,63]

- **Avoid saturated fats**, which can increase inflammation (a known cause of cancer), particularly if you're post-menopausal.[64]

- There is disagreement in the medical community about the benefits or detriments of **soy.** A recent Chinese study suggested that soy might reduce recurrence in all breast cancer patients, but other medical studies are concerned that for women with estrogen-responsive cancer, soy might increase risk. It appears low doses of soy might act like an anti-estrogen and reduce risk, and high doses of soy might increase risk.[65]

- The jury is still out on whether **vitamins** can be helpful in preventing cancer, or whether it's better for you to get your nutritional needs through food alone. Ask your doctor.[66]

- Ask your doctor about taking **aspirin**, which has been shown to inhibit breast cancer metastasis.[67]

- **Drink less wine**. According to a study at The Dana-Farber Cancer Institute, even modest levels of alcohol consumption—as little as one alcoholic drink each day—can increase risk of breast cancer. Those who consume 3-6 glasses of wine each week are 15% more likely to be diagnosed with breast cancer. Those drinking fewer than three drinks a week show no increased risk.[69]

- Needless to say, getting your nutrition and exercise into shape, while continue to engage in smoking, drinking, or drugs, is somewhat pointless. Commit, right now, to overhauling your health, whatever that might mean.

Checklist: Menu Planning

✓	Menu Planning
☐	Start by organizing your favorite recipes that meet your cancer diet guidelines and compiling them in one binder so you (or someone else) can easily cook from them.
☐	Compile a grocery shopping list for each week around the meals that you plan to make. (See p. 92)
☐	Begin cooking and freezing meals that you and your family will want to eat post-surgery. Carefully label and date the dishes so you know what they are (and when they were frozen), and keep a list taped to the outside of the freezer so you know exactly which and how many meals you have.
☐	Gather take-out menus from your favorite (healthy) restaurants (take two from each), and mark what you typically order. Tape one set to your refrigerator, so that in a pinch your family and helpful friends can order what you'll want; put another set with your hospital bag, in case you need to send out for emergency supplies for your family at home while you're in the hospital post-surgery.

Sample Weekly Menu

Remember to focus on whole grains, fish, and vegetables:

Sample Weekly Menu		
	Lunch	**Dinner**
Sunday	Vegetable lasagna	Salmon with kale
Monday	Caesar salad	Tuna Nicoise
Tuesday	Humus wraps	Vegetable stir fry
Wednesday	Greek salad	Grilled salmon
Thursday	Sardine sandwiches	Brown rice sushi
Friday	Whole wheat sesame noodles	BBQ salmon
Saturday	Poached salmon	Vegetable lo mein

Here is a blank menu chart for you to record your own weekly menu. You can also find a menu chart in the appendix on p. 291.

Weekly Menu For _____		
	Lunch	**Dinner**
Sunday		
Monday		
Tuesday		
Wednesday		
Thursday		
Friday		
Saturday		

Shopping List

Here is a sample shopping list you can photocopy, keep on your refrigerator, and just circle what you need:

Shopping List		
Produce		**Spices**
Apples	Mushrooms-maitake	Anise
Apricots	Mushrooms-shiitake	Basil
Asparagus	Mushrooms-reishi	Bay leaves
Avocadoes	Onions	Black pepper
Banana	Oranges	Cardamom
Berries	Parsley	Cayenne pepper
Broccoli	Parsnips	Cilantro
Cabbage (green)	Peaches	Cinnamon
Cabbage (red)	Pears	Cloves
Carrots	Peppers	Coriander
Cauliflower	Pineapple	Cumin
Celery	Plums	Curry powder
Collard greens	Pomegranates	Dill
Cucumbers	Pumpkins	Fennel
Eggplants	Radishes	Ginger
Garlic	Raspberries	Nutmeg
Ginger root	Red onions	Oregano
Grapes	Scallions	Paprika
Kale	Squash	Parsley
Lemons	String beans	Red pepper
Lettuce	Sweet potatoes	Rosemary
Limes	Tomatoes	Tarragon
Melons	Watercress	Thyme
	Zucchini	Turmeric

Nuts/Seeds

Almonds
Chestnuts
Flax seed
Peanuts
Pecans
Pine nuts
Pumpkin seeds
Sesame seeds
Sunflower seeds
Walnuts

Beverages

Bottled water
Seltzer

Canned

Applesauce
Crushed tomatoes
Herring
Mackerel
Olives
Salmon
Sardines
Spaghetti sauce
Tomato paste
Tuna (canned)

Fresh fish

Household

Aluminum foil
Dish soap
Garbage bags
Kleenex
Laundry detergent
Napkins
Paper cups
Paper plates
Saran Wrap
Toilet paper
Toothpaste

Baking

Baking powder
Baking soda
Cocoa powder
Whole wheat flour
Whole wheat pastry
Yeast

Grains/Pasta

Barley
Bulgur wheat
Brown rice
Cereal-whole grain
Oatmeal (whole oats)
Whole couscous
Whole wheat bagels
Whole wheat bread
Whole wheat pasta

Beans

Aduki beans
Black beans
Chickpeas
Kidney beans
Lentils
Pinto beans
Split peas

Other

Coffee
Green tea
Humus
Olive oil
Salt
Sesame oil
Vinegar
Whole-wheat crackers

Seaweed

Arame
Dulse
Hijiki
Kelp
Kombu
Nori
Wakame

Other items needed this week:

Exercise Overview

- There is evidence that exercise reduces breast cancer risk: the Women's Health Initiative study showed that even 1½ hours of walking per week reduced risk by 18%. The American Cancer Society recommends 45-60 minutes of exercise per day.

- Exercise can alleviate side-effects of cancer treatment.

- Exercise can also alleviate cancer treatment fatigue, experienced by a majority of women.

- Many cancer patients don't feel up to their usual workouts, but a long walk every day, 20 minutes of yoga and stretching, or even meditating, can be helpful in the absence of more rigorous exercise.

- If you find it difficult to stick to an exercise plan even in your normal life, then commit yourself to exercise by involving someone else: Take a class, or arrange walking dates with different friends on different days.

Diet References

The *Diet Suggestions* section of this chapter was based on over 500 published medical studies linking nutrition to cancer. A selection of these references is included here for medical professionals and others interested in learning more.

[1] *The role of dietary factors in cancer prevention: beyond fruits and vegetables*, Williams MT, Hord NG, Nutr Clin Pract. 2005 Aug;20(4):451-9, www.ncbi.nlm.nih.gov/pubmed/16207684

[2] *Why whole grains are protective: biological mechanisms*, Slavin J, Proc Nutr Soc. 2003 Feb;62(1):129-34, www.ncbi.nlm.nih.gov/pubmed/12740067

[3] *Session: whole cereal grains, fibre and human cancer wholegrain cereals and cancer in Italy*, La Vecchia C, Chatenoud L, Negri E, Franceschi S, Proc Nutr Soc. 2003 Feb;62(1):45-9, www.ncbi.nlm.nih.gov/pubmed/12740056

[4] *Dietary carotenoids and vitamins A, C, and E and risk of breast cancer*, Zhang S, Hunter DJ, Forman MR, Rosner BA, Speizer FE, Colditz GA, Manson JE, Hankinson SE, Willett WC, J Natl Cancer Inst. 1999 Mar 17;91(6):547-56, www.ncbi.nlm.nih.gov/pubmed/10088626

[5] *Retinoids, carotenoids, and human breast cancer cell cultures: a review of differential effects*, Prakash P, Krinsky NI, Russell RM, Nutr Rev. 2000 Jun;58(6):170-6, www.ncbi.nlm.nih.gov/pubmed/10885324

[6] *Dietary cod protein restores insulin-induced activation of phosphatidylinositol 3-kinase/Akt and GLUT4 translocation to the T-tubules in skeletal muscle of high-fat-fed obese rats*, Tremblay F, Lavigne C, Jacques H, Marette A, Diabetes. 2003 Jan;52(1):29-37, www.ncbi.nlm.nih.gov/pubmed/12502490

[7] *Antioxidant and antiproliferative activities of common fruits*, Sun J, Chu YF, Wu X, Liu RH, J Agric Food Chem. 2002 Dec 4;50(25):7449-54, www.ncbi.nlm.nih.gov/pubmed/12452674

[8] *Fruit, vegetables, and the prevention of cancer: research challenges*, Temple NJ, Gladwin KK, Nutrition. 2003 May;19(5):467-70, www.ncbi.nlm.nih.gov/pubmed/12714102

[9] *What is the nutrition and lifestyle profile in oncology patients? Cross-sectional study*, Rolão A, Monteiro-Grillo I, Camilo ME, Ravasco P, Acta Med Port. 2011 Dec;24 Suppl 2:113-22. Epub 2011 Dec 31, www.ncbi.nlm.nih.gov/pubmed/22849894

[10] *Meat consumption and cancer risk: a case-control study in Uruguay,* Aune D, De Stefani E, Ronco A, Boffetta P, Deneo-Pellegrini H, Acosta G, Mendilaharsu M, Asian Pac J Cancer Prev. 2009 Jul-Sep;10(3):429-36, www.ncbi.nlm.nih.gov/pubmed/19640186

[11] *Nutrition and breast cancer risk by age 50: a population-based case-control study in Germany,* Hermann S, Linseisen J, Chang-Claude J, Nutr Cancer. 2002;44(1):23-34, www.ncbi.nlm.nih.gov/pubmed/12672638

[12] *Dietary patterns and the risk of postmenopausal breast cancer*, Fung TT, Hu FB, Holmes MD, Rosner BA, Hunter DJ, Colditz GA, Willett WC, Int J Cancer. 2005 Aug 10;116(1):116-21, www.ncbi.nlm.nih.gov/pubmed/15756679

[13] *Nutrition-related issues for the breast cancer survivor*, Demark-Wahnefried W, Rock CL, Semin Oncol. 2003 Dec;30(6):789-98, www.ncbi.nlm.nih.gov/pubmed/14663779

[14] *Dairy foods and risk of breast cancer: a case-control study in Montevideo, Uruguay,* Ronco AL, De Stéfani E, Dáttoli R, Eur J Cancer Prev. 2002 Oct;11(5):457-63, www.ncbi.nlm.nih.gov/pubmed/12394243

[15] *Diet and cancer in Mediterranean countries: carbohydrates and fats,* Bosetti C, Pelucchi C, La Vecchia C, Public Health Nutr. 2009 Sep;12(9A):1595-600, www.ncbi.nlm.nih.gov/pubmed/19689827

[16] *ACS Guidelines on Nutrition and Physical Activity for Cancer Prevention,* www.cancer.org/Healthy/EatHealthyGetActive/ ACSGuidelinesonNutritionPhysicalActivityforCancerPrevention/acs-guidelines-on-nutrition-and-physical-activity-for-cancer-prevention-summary

[17] *ACS Guidelines on Nutrition and Physical Activity for Cancer Prevention,* www.cancer.org/Healthy/EatHealthyGetActive/ ACSGuidelinesonNutritionPhysicalActivityforCancerPrevention/acs-guidelines-on-nutrition-and-physical-activity-for-cancer-prevention-common-questions

[18] *Consumption of sweet foods and breast cancer risk in Italy*, Tavani A, Giordano L, Gallus S, Talamini R, Franceschi S, Giacosa A, Montella M, La Vecchia C, Ann Oncol. 2006 Feb;17(2):341-345, annonc.oxfordjournals.org/content/17/2/341

[19] *Dietary glycemic index and glycemic load and breast cancer risk in the European Prospective Investigation into Cancer and Nutrition (EPIC),* Romieu I, Ferrari P, Rinaldi S, Slimani N, Jenab M, Olsen A, Tjonneland A, Overvad K, Boutron-Ruault MC, Lajous M, Kaaks R, Teucher B, Boeing H, Trichopoulou A, Naska A, Vasilopoulo E, Sacerdote C,

Tumino R, Masala G, Sieri S, Panico S, Bueno-de-Mesquita HB, Van-der-A D, van Gils CH, Peeters PH, Lund E, Skeie G, Asli LA, Rodriguez L, Navarro C, Amiano P, Sanchez MJ, Barricarte A, Buckland G, Sonestedt E, Wirfält E, Hallmans G, Johansson I, Key TJ, Allen NE, Khaw KT, Wareham NJ, Norat T, Riboli E, Clavel-Chapelon F, Am J Clin Nutr. 2012 Aug;96(2):345-55, www.ncbi.nlm.nih.gov/pubmed/22760570

[20] *Dietary walnut suppressed mammary gland tumorigenesis in the C(3)1 TAg mouse*, Hardman WE, Ion G, Akinsete JA, Witte TR, Nutr Cancer. 2011;63(6):960-70, www.ncbi.nlm.nih.gov/pubmed/21774594

[21] *Diet and breast cancer: the possible connection with sugar consumption*, Seely S, Horrobin DF, Med Hypotheses. 1983 Jul;11(3):319-27, www.ncbi.nlm.nih.gov/pubmed/6645999

[22] *Apigenin prevents development of medroxyprogesterone acetate-accelerated 7,12-dimethylbenz(a)anthracene-induced mammary tumors in Sprague-Dawley rats*, Mafuvadze B, Benakanakere I, López Pérez FR, Besch-Williford C, Ellersieck MR, Hyder SM, Cancer Prev Res (Phila). 2011 Aug;4(8):1316-24, www.ncbi.nlm.nih.gov/pubmed/21505181

[23] *Dietary patterns differ between urban and rural older, long-term survivors of breast, prostate, and colorectal cancer and are associated with body mass index*, Miller PE, Morey MC, Hartman TJ, Snyder DC, Sloane R, Cohen HJ, Demark-Wahnefried W, J Acad Nutr Diet. 2012 Jun;112(6):824-31, 831.e1, www.ncbi.nlm.nih.gov/pubmed/22709810

[24] *Coffee consumption modifies risk of estrogen-receptor negative breast cancer*, Li J, Seibold P, Chang-Claude J, Flesch-Janys D, Liu J, Czene K, Humphreys K, Hall P, Breast Cancer Res. 2011 May 14;13(3):R49, www.ncbi.nlm.nih.gov/sites/entrez/21569535

[25] *Joint effects of dietary vitamin D and sun exposure on breast cancer risk: results from the French E3N cohort*, Engel P, Fagherazzi G, Mesrine S, Boutron-Ruault MC, Clavel-Chapelon F, Cancer Epidemiol Biomarkers Prev. 2011 Jan;20(1):187-98, www.ncbi.nlm.nih.gov/pubmed/21127286

[26] *Olive oil, an essential component of the Mediterranean diet, and breast cancer*, Escrich E, Moral R, Solanas M, Public Health Nutr. 2011 Dec;14(12A):2323-32, www.ncbi.nlm.nih.gov/pubmed/22166191

[27] *Sulforaphane, a dietary component of broccoli/broccoli sprouts, inhibits breast cancer stem cells*, Li Y, Zhang T, Korkaya H, Liu S, Lee HF, Newman B, Yu Y, Clouthier SG, Schwartz SJ, Wicha MS, Sun D, Clin Cancer Res. 2010 May 1;16(9):2580-90, www.ncbi.nlm.nih.gov/pubmed/20388854

[28] *Flight attendants, breast cancer, and melatonin*, Barker ME, Stookey JD, Lancet 1998 Oct;352(9137):1389, www.thelancet.com/journals/lancet/article/PIIS0140-6736(05)60784-2/fulltext

[29] *Angiogenesis inhibited by drinking tea*, Cao Y, Cao R, Nature 1999 Apr;398(6726):381, www.nature.com/nature/journal/v398/n6726/abs/398381a0.html

[30] *Green tea and tea polyphenols in cancer prevention*, Chen D, Daniel KG, Kuhn DJ, Kazi A, Bhuiyan M, Li L, Wang Z, Wan SB, Lam WH, Chan TH, Dou QP, Front Biosci. 2004 Sep 1;9:2618-31, www.ncbi.nlm.nih.gov/pubmed/15358585

[31] *Lycopene*, www.cancer.org/Treatment/TreatmentsandSideEffects/ ComplementaryandAlternativeMedicine/DietandNutrition/lycopene

[32] *Lycopene, beta-carotene, and colorectal adenomas*, Erhardt JG, Meisner C, Bode JC, Bode C, Am J Clin Nutr. 2003 Dec;78(6):1219-24, www.ncbi.nlm.nih.gov/pubmed/ 14668286

[33] *Does gamma-tocopherol play a role in the primary prevention of heart disease and cancer? A review*, Dietrich M, Traber MG, Jacques PF, Cross CE, Hu Y, Block G, J Am Coll Nutr. 2006 Aug;25(4):292-9, www.ncbi.nlm.nih.gov/pubmed/16943450

[34] *Urinary isothiocyanate levels, brassica, and human breast cancer*, Fowke JH, Chung FL, Jin F, Qi D, Cai Q, Conaway C, Cheng JR, Shu XO, Gao YT, Zheng W, Cancer Res. 2003 Jul 15;63(14):3980-6, www.ncbi.nlm.nih.gov/pubmed/12873994

[35] *Brassica vegetables and breast cancer risk*, Terry P, Wolk A, Persson I, Magnusson C, JAMA. 2001 Jun 20;285(23):2975-7, www.ncbi.nlm.nih.gov/pubmed/11410091

[36] *Raw and cooked vegetables, fruits, selected micronutrients, and breast cancer risk: a case-control study in Germany*, Adzersen KH, Jess P, Freivogel KW, Gerhard I, Bastert G, Nutr Cancer. 2003;46(2):131-7, www.ncbi.nlm.nih.gov/pubmed/14690788

[37] *Combinations of tomato and broccoli enhance antitumor activity in dunning r3327-h prostate adenocarcinomas*, Canene-Adams K, Lindshield BL, Wang S, Jeffery EH, Clinton SK, Erdman JW Jr, Cancer Res. 2007 Jan 15;67(2):836-43. Epub 2007 Jan 9, www.ncbi.nlm.nih.gov/pubmed/17213256

[38] *Dietary intake of vitamin K and risk of prostate cancer in the Heidelberg cohort of the European Prospective Investigation into Cancer and Nutrition (EPIC-Heidelberg)*, Nimptsch K, Rohrmann S, Linseisen J, Am J Clin Nutr. 2008 Apr;87(4):985-92, www.ncbi.nlm.nih.gov/pubmed/18400723

[39] *Specialty Supplements and Breast Cancer Risk in the VITamins And Lifestyle (VITAL) Cohort,* Brasky TM, Lampe JW, Potter JD, Patterson RE, White E, Cancer Epidemiol Biomarkers Prev. 2010 Jul;19(7)1696-708, cebp.aacrjournals.org/content/19/7/1696

[40] *Flavonoids and breast cancer risk in Italy,* Bosetti C, Spertini L, Parpinel M, Gnagnarella P, Lagiou P, Negri E, Franceschi S, Montella M, Peterson J, Dwyer J, Giacosa A, La Vecchia C, Cancer Epidemiol Biomarkers Prev. 2005 Apr;14(4):805-8, www.ncbi.nlm.nih.gov/pubmed/15824147

[41] *Quercetin,* www.cancer.org/Treatment/TreatmentsandSideEffects/ComplementaryandAlternativeMedicine/DietandNutrition/quercetin

[42] *Onion and garlic use and human cancer,* Galeone C, Pelucchi C, Levi F, Negri E, Franceschi S, Talamini R, Giacosa A, La Vecchia C, Am J Clin Nutr. 2006 Nov;84(5):1027-32, www.ncbi.nlm.nih.gov/pubmed/17093154

[43] *Shiitake Mushroom,* www.cancer.org/Treatment/TreatmentsandSideEffects/ComplementaryandAlternativeMedicine/DietandNutrition/shiitake-mushroom

[44] *About Herbs, Botanicals & Other Products: Shiitake Mushroom,* www.mskcc.org/cancer-care/herb/shiitake-mushroom

[45] *Suppression of the nuclear factor-kappaB activation pathway by spice-derived phytochemicals: reasoning for seasoning,* Aggarwal BB, Shishodia S, Ann N Y Acad Sci. 2004 Dec;1030:434-41, www.ncbi.nlm.nih.gov/pubmed/15659827

[46] *Phase I clinical trial of curcumin, a chemopreventive agent, in patients with high-risk or pre-malignant lesions,* Cheng AL, Hsu CH, Lin JK, Hsu MM, Ho YF, Shen TS, Ko JY, Lin JT, Lin BR, Ming-Shiang W, Yu HS, Jee SH, Chen GS, Chen TM, Chen CA, Lai MK, Pu YS, Pan MH, Wang YJ, Tsai CC, Hsieh CY, Anticancer Res. 2001 Jul-Aug;21(4B):2895-900, www.ncbi.nlm.nih.gov/pubmed/11712783

[47] *Dietary cardamom inhibits the formation of azoxymethane-induced aberrant crypt foci in mice and reduces COX-2 and iNOS expression in the colon,* Sengupta A, Ghosh S, Bhattacharjee S, Asian Pac J Cancer Prev. 2005 Apr-Jun;6(2):118-22, www.ncbi.nlm.nih.gov/pubmed/16101317

[48] *Pharmacology of rosemary (Rosmarinus officinalis Linn.) and its therapeutic potentials,* al-Sereiti MR, Abu-Amer KM, Sen P, Indian J Exp Biol. 1999 Feb;37(2):124-30, www.ncbi.nlm.nih.gov/pubmed/10641130

[49] *Ginger Root Supplement Reduced Colon Inflammation Markers,* www.aacr.org/home/public--media/aacr-in-the-news.aspx?d=2498%20

[50] *Health benefits of nuts: potential role of antioxidants*, Blomhoff R, Carlsen MH, Andersen LF, Jacobs DR Jr, Br J Nutr. 2006 Nov;96 Suppl 2:S52-60, www.ncbi.nlm.nih.gov/pubmed/17125534

[51] *Phytochemical composition of nuts*, Chen CY, Blumberg JB, Asia Pac J Clin Nutr. 2008;17 Suppl 1:329-32, www.ncbi.nlm.nih.gov/pubmed/18296370

[52] Prevention and therapy of cancer by dietary monoterpenes, Crowell PL, J Nutr. 1999 Mar;129(3):775S-778S, www.ncbi.nlm.nih.gov/pubmed/10082788

[53] *A comparative study of the anti-inflammatory, anticoagulant, antiangiogenic, and antiadhesive activities of nine different fucoidans from brown seaweeds*, Cumashi A, Ushakova NA, Preobrazhenskaya ME, D'Incecco A, Piccoli A, Totani L, Tinari N, Morozevich GE, Berman AE, Bilan MI, Usov AI, Ustyuzhanina NE, Grachev AA, Sanderson CJ, Kelly M, Rabinovich GA, Iacobelli S, Nifantiev NE; Consorzio Interuniversitario Nazionale per la Bio-Oncologia, Italy, Glycobiology. 2007 May;17(5):541-52. Epub 2007 Feb 12, www.ncbi.nlm.nih.gov/pubmed/17296677

[54] *In vivo modulation of 4E binding protein 1 (4E-BP1) phosphorylation by watercress: a pilot study*, Alwi SSS, Cavell B, Telang U, Morris ME, Parry BM, Packham G, Brit J of Nutrition. 2010 Nov;104(9):1288-96, journals.cambridge.org/action/displayAbstract?fromPage=online&aid=7918284

[55] *Ellagitannin-rich pomegranate extract inhibits angiogenesis in prostate cancer in vitro and in vivo*, Sartippour MR, Seeram NP, Rao JY, Moro A, Harris DM, Henning SM, Firouzi A, Rettig MB, Aronson WJ, Pantuck AJ, Heber D, Int J Oncol. 2008 Feb;32(2):475-80, www.ncbi.nlm.nih.gov/pubmed/18202771

[56] *Chemoprevention of Esophageal Tumorigenesis by Dietary Administration of Lyophilized Black Raspberries*, Kresty LA, Morse MA, Morgan C, Carlton PS, Lu J, Gupta A, Blackwood M, Stoner GD, Cancer Res. 2001 Aug;61(16):6112-9, cancerres.aacrjournals.org/content/61/16/6112

[57] *Bromelain*, www.cancer.org/Treatment/TreatmentsandSideEffects/ComplementaryandAlternativeMedicine/HerbsVitaminsandMinerals/bromelain

[58] *Pentameric procyanidin from Theobroma cacao selectively inhibits growth of human breast cancer cells*, Ramljak D, Romanczyk LJ, Metheny-Barlow LJ, Thompson N, Knezevic V, Galperin M, Ramesh A, Dickson RB, Mol Cancer Ther. 2005 Apr;4(4):537-46, www.ncbi.nlm.nih.gov/pubmed/15827326

[59] *Dietary phytoestrogen intake—lignans and isoflavones—and breast cancer risk (Canada)*, Cotterchio M, Boucher BA, Kreiger N, Mills CA, Thompson LU, Cancer Causes Control. 2008 Apr;19(3):259-72, www.ncbi.nlm.nih.gov/pubmed/17992574

[60] *Lignans and breast cancer risk in pre- and post-menopausal women: meta-analyses of observational studies*, Velentzis LS, Cantwell MM, Cardwell C, Keshtgar MR, Leathem AJ, Woodside JV, Br J Cancer. 2009 May 5;100(9):1492-8, www.ncbi.nlm.nih.gov/pubmed/ 19337250

[61] *Pilot study of dietary fat restriction and flaxseed supplementation in men with prostate cancer before surgery: exploring the effects on hormonal levels, prostate-specific antigen, and histopathologic features*, Demark-Wahnefried W, Price DT, Polascik TJ, Robertson CN, Anderson EE, Paulson DF, Walther PJ, Gannon M, Vollmer RT, Urology. 2001 Jul;58(1):47-52, www.ncbi.nlm.nih.gov/pubmed/11445478

[62] Dietary lignan intake and postmenopausal breast cancer risk by estrogen and progesterone receptor status, Touillaud MS, Thiébaut AC, Fournier A, Niravong M, Boutron-Ruault MC, Clavel-Chapelon F, J Natl Cancer Inst. 2007 Mar 21;99(6):475-86, www.ncbi.nlm.nih.gov/pubmed/17374837

[63] *Mediterranean diet and health: biological importance of olive oil*, Alarcón de la Lastra C, Barranco MD, Motilva V, Herrerías JM, Curr Pharm Des. 2001 Jul;7(10):933-50, www.ncbi.nlm.nih.gov/pubmed/11472248

[64] *Dietary fat and breast cancer risk in the European Prospective Investigation into Cancer and Nutrition*, Sieri S, Krogh V, Ferrari P, Berrino F, Pala V, Thiébaut AC, Tjønneland A, Olsen A, Overvad K, Jakobsen MU, Clavel-Chapelon F, Chajes V, Boutron-Ruault MC, Kaaks R, Linseisen J, Boeing H, Nöthlings U, Trichopoulou A, Naska A, Lagiou P, Panico S, Palli D, Vineis P, Tumino R, Lund E, Kumle M, Skeie G, González CA, Ardanaz E, Amiano P, Tormo MJ, Martínez-García C, Quirós JR, Berglund G, Gullberg B, Hallmans G, Lenner P, Bueno-de-Mesquita HB, van Duijnhoven FJ, Peeters PH, van Gils CH, Key TJ, Crowe FL, Bingham S, Khaw KT, Rinaldi S, Slimani N, Jenab M, Norat T, Riboli E, Am J Clin Nutr. 2008 Nov;88(5):1304-12, www.ncbi.nlm.nih.gov/pubmed/18996867

[65] *Soy food intake after diagnosis of breast cancer and survival: an in-depth analysis of combined evidence from cohort studies of US and Chinese women*, Nechuta SJ, Caan BJ, Chen WY, Lu W, Chen Z, Kwan ML, Flatt SW, Zheng Y, Zheng W, Pierce JP, Shu XO, Am J Clin Nutr. 2012 Jul;96(1):123-32, www.ncbi.nlm.nih.gov/pubmed/22648714

[66] *Multivitamin use and breast cancer outcomes in women with early-stage breast cancer: the Life After Cancer Epidemiology study*, Kwan ML, Greenlee H, Lee VS, Castillo A, Gunderson EP, Habel LA, Kushi LH, Sweeney C, Tam EK, Caan BJ, Breast Cancer Res Treat. 2011 Nov;130(1):195-205, www.ncbi.nlm.nih.gov/pubmed/21559824

[67] *Aspirin intake and survival after breast cancer*, Holmes MD, Chen WY, Li L, Hertzmark E, Spiegelman D, Hankinson SE, J Clin Oncol. 2010 Mar 20;28(9):1467-72, www.ncbi.nlm.nih.gov/pubmed/20159825

[68] *Dietary intakes of mushrooms and green tea combine to reduce the risk of breast cancer in Chinese women*, Zhang M, Huang J, Xie X, Holman CD, Int J Cancer. 2009 Mar 15;124(6):1404-8, www.ncbi.nlm.nih.gov/pubmed/19048616

[69] *Moderate alcohol consumption during adult life, drinking patterns, and breast cancer risk*, Chen WY, Rosner B, Hankinson SE, Colditz GA, Willett WC, JAMA. 2011 Nov 2;306(17):1884-90, www.ncbi.nlm.nih.gov/pubmed/22045766

Day 5:
Shopping for Equipment

ༀ ༚

You can make your life easier, during and post-treatment, by purchasing in advance the equipment you're likely to need. (Better yet, give some friends the list and let them help you shop.) Here's a list of what most women find useful; whenever possible, we've offered suggestions of online sources for these products, so that you can shop from home.

Checklist: Products and Purchases

✓	Products and Purchases
☐	**Drainage tube solutions.** Immediately post-surgery, you'll need a convenient way to accommodate one to four (sometimes more) drainage tubes attached to your chest. Here are several options. (If your insurance will cover the costs, save receipts.)
	• You can use safety pins.
	• You can use a piece of thick ribbon, long enough to knot around your neck (extending to mid-chest) so that you can have an anchor from which to

dangle your drainage tubes; this will make showering much easier. (Or snag one of your spouse's unused ties, which will work just as well.)

- You can buy a drain bulb holder for about $20. *PromedicsProducts.com/?110010*

- You can buy Peel-and-stick Pockets, which adhere to your clothing and will hold drainage tubes ($20 for pack of five). *www.Pink-Pockets.com*

- For about $40 you can get shorts that accommodate the drains (but these may make it tricky to use the bathroom). *www.SurgiShorts .com/surgishort/surgi-shorts*

- For about $60 you can get a pocket camisole (*www.SofteeUSA.com/home/st1/page_268*) that hides the drainage bulbs. (The camisole will also hide whatever prosthesis you end up using, so it can double as a mastectomy camisole.) You may want to buy two, so that you have one to wash and one to wear. If you'll be having lymph nodes removed and will find pulling the camisole over your head too challenging, you can buy front-closure camisoles (but some women complain that these are uncomfortable because they're too tight-fitting): *www.WomansPersonalHealth.com/ amoena-mastectomy-camisole*

☐	**Loose button-up shirts.** If you'll be having chemotherapy, and your doctor has decided that you should have an infusion port, you'll want a few button-up shirts so that the nurses can easily access your port to attach the IV. You can use any button-up shirt for this purpose, but make sure you have a few in your closet; pullovers don't work nearly as well. You'll also want a loose button-up shirt (or two) to wear immediately post-surgery, when it's difficult to pull shirts on over your head.
☐	**Loose pants.** If you're having immediate reconstruction TRAM flap surgery, purchase some loose-fitting, oversized cotton snap pants so that your pants won't pull on your scar.
☐	**Pull-on slippers.** Make sure you have a pair of slip-on slippers and/or shoes, because it will be uncomfortable to bend over to tie on shoes. Footwear with a grip on the sole will help you avoid slipping.
☐	**Sports bra.** If you're getting a lumpectomy, be sure to buy a sports bra; you'll probably be instructed to wear a bra (even at night) for the first few days after surgery, and then during the day for the next two weeks. Consider a bra that hooks in the front, because it will be challenging to hook a bra behind you in the first days post-surgery. JC Penney offers an Underscore Zip Front cotton sports bra for $15: *JCPenny.com*, item number is RN128-0107Q;

	JustMySize.com offers a Valmont Zip Front Sports Bra (style 20357) for plus sizes.
☐	**Underwire bra.** If you're having immediate reconstruction, ask your plastic surgeon if he recommends an underwire bra. Some surgeons advise wearing these 24/7 for 3-4 months, immediately after the drainage tubes are removed. Women advise an unlined bra devoid of center trim, so that it does not push the implants out to the side. In addition, the band and straps should fit quite snugly, and the wire should encapsulate the implants completely, with the center wires slightly away from your chest and not touching the implants themselves. You can find Chatelle, Fantasie, Freya, Le Mystere, Soma, and Wacoal bras at: • *www.HerRoom.com* • *www.BareNecessities.com* • *www.BiggerBras.com* • *shop.Nordstrom.com* • *www.BraSmyth.com*
☐	**Knitted Knockers.** Eventually you may want a more fitted prosthesis, but surgeons recommend waiting at least three or four weeks, until your surgical scars heal. So as an interim measure, rather than baring your now-flat chest to the world, put a 'knitted knocker' into your camisole pocket for coverage. Some women find these so comfortable that they

	become a permanent solution. *TheKnittingExperience.com/knitted_knockers_program* offers them free to breast cancer survivors; email them at *info@TheKnittingExperience.com*. You can purchase more at *TitBits.ca/v1/tb_shop.html*.
☐	**Mastectomy camisoles.** Plan to buy yourself at least one or two camisoles to accommodate your knitted knockers or prostheses as a stop-gap, even if you're eventually planning on reconstruction. (You can also use your drainage tube camisole, but usually these get a little mucked up during the month of intensive use right after surgery.) • *www.TLCDirect.org* • *www.SofteeUSA.com* • *StillYou.com/Products/tanktop.html*
☐	**Guided visualization tape.** You'll probably benefit from doing your own personalized, guided visualization tape for use before and during your surgery (see p. 139).
☐	**Comfy clothing.** You'll want at least one very comfortable outfit that you can throw on every week to wear to chemotherapy. It should include a button-down shirt (to accommodate your infusion port if you'll have one), a comfortable jacket to guard against hospital chill, snuggly socks, and shoes that are

☐	comfortable enough to sleep in (because you may be there for several hours.)
☐	**Wig or headscarf.** Before you lose your hair, figure out whether you'll be happier in a wig or some sort of scarf or hat, and buy in advance. The cost of a wig may be covered by your insurance. (For insurance purposes, the wig is a 'cranial prosthesis.') Your local American Cancer Society office may offer free wigs; check with them before buying. There are literally hundreds of places online (and off) to buy wigs and scarves; here are just a few: • Chemo Comforts, *www.ChemoComforts.com* • Chemo Savvy, (888) 599-3560, *www.ChemoSavvy.com* • Headcovers, (800) 264-4287, *www.Headcovers.com* • Look of Love, (800) 526-7627, *www.LookOfLove.com*
☐	An inexpensive **disposable cell phone** so that you don't have to worry about your pricey cell phone being stolen in the hospital.
☐	**Soft cap.** If you'll be doing chemotherapy, get a warm, soft cap in which you can sleep comfortably; bald can be cold. If you can find a cap that is seam-free, it will be more comfortable. (Lands End, *www.*

	LandsEnd.com, and L.L. Bean, *www.LLBean.com*, both offer fuzzy caps made of polar fleece available online, *Headscarves.com* offers $18 polar-fleece bandanas.)
☐	**Thank-you notes.** You will have many people who do wonderful things for you all during your treatment. Be sure you're stocked up on thank you notes (and a pen you enjoy using, and stamps, and a current address book) so that you can easily thank people.
☐	**Moisturizer.** Most people in treatment for chemotherapy end up with dry skin; using a moisturizer helps. Moisturizing your arms consistently also can help prevent lymphedema. Buy a lotion without fragrance, because you'll likely be hyper-sensitive to smells during chemotherapy.
☐	**Eyebrow pencil.** During chemotherapy, most women end up losing not only their scalp hair but also their eyebrows, and often their eyelashes as well. Having an eyebrow pencil ready so that you can draw on your brows will help you feel less vulnerable. The glue in fake eyelashes can cause infections, so just use a dark eyeliner pencil around your eyes, and skip the falsies.
☐	**EMLA and Tegaderm.** If you're getting an infusion port implanted for chemotherapy, ask whether the hospital will supply EMLA and Tegaderm; if not, buy some yourself. Applying EMLA to the port site (and holding it in place with the Tegaderm adhesive) will partially anesthetize the skin so that the IV insertion is

☐	less painful.
☐	**Facemask.** If you're worried about germs during chemotherapy, buy an inexpensive nose-mask to limit germs, and wear it in public places.
☐	**Rubber gloves.** Buy inexpensive rubber gloves to use when washing dishes and other household chores, to prevent infection (and possible lymphedema).
☐	**Alcohol antibiotic hand sanitizer.** Keep sanitizer in all your bathrooms and near the doors of your home to encourage guests to shed unwelcome germs at the door.
☐	Make sure you have/buy **gauze** and sanitary pads if you're having immediate reconstruction—you may need absorbent material for leaks.
☐	**Throat lozenges.** During surgery you'll have had a tube down your throat, so your throat may feel scratchy and uncomfortable afterwards; lozenges or Xylocaine Viscous (lidocaine viscous) can help.
☐	**Biotene.** Available as toothpaste, mouthwash, or chewing gum, Biotene prevents chemotherapy mouth sores. Peridex is also effective.
☐	**Baby aspirin.** Since cancer is a disease of inflammation, many women take low-dose (81 mg) baby aspirin (one per day). (Be sure not to take aspirin for the weeks immediately before and after

☐	surgery, since aspirin can affect blood clotting.)
☐	**Sanitary wipes.** Carry these around with you in case you need to sterilize things, or to use instead of communal or public towels in restrooms, etc. and plan to disseminate them through your house as needed.
☐	**New glasses.** Chemotherapy will dry out your eyes, so if you wear contact lenses, consider getting an updated pair of prescription glasses for the duration.
☐	**Pain relief.** Whether it's for the pain of surgery, or the bone pain many women feel along with their Neulastim (Neulasta, Imupeg, pegfilgrastim) injections, have a supply of painkiller on hand.
☐	**Seasick bands.** Though chemotherapy is continually improving, many women still experience nausea. Try getting accupressure (seasick) wrist-bands; some women find that these help their nausea.
☐	**Deodorant substitute.** If you're going to get radiation, your doctor may discourage your use of deodorant because the trace metals can irritate your skin. Good substitutes for regular deodorant include cornstarch, Tom's of Maine products, and Arm & Hammer Baking Soda.
☐	**Aloe vera or Bag Balm.** When radiation irritates your skin, some women use aloe vera plants (just slit the leaf and slather the liquid over the radiation site) or

	Bag Balm (found in pharmacies and farm stores). Aquaphor and Eucerin also work. But check with your radiation oncologist first to make sure these won't affect your treatment.
☐	**Vitamin E.** When your hair begins to fall out during chemotherapy, many women find it's easier to just shave it all off, rather than continuing to watch it fall out in clumps. If your scalp still feels itchy or irritated, rubbing vitamin E over it might help. Women also use vitamin E on surgery scars for smoother recovery; ask your doctor.
☐	**Mastectomy pillow.** After a bilateral mastectomy, if sleeping on your back (the only possible position) proves uncomfortable; a mastectomy pillow may be helpful. • *www.MakeMeHeal.com/mmh/product/ mastectomy/pillows/index.vm?procid=33& catid=440* • *MyComfortQuest.com*
☐	**Scottevest.** If you're at risk of lymphedema, you'll be told not to carry a purse for the foreseeable future (and possibly forever). But most women find a purse-like substitute essential. Scottevest (*www.Scottevest .com*) offers a great solution: Vests (and jackets) with lots of pockets which allow you to absorb the weight across your shoulders and back, rather than on your now-compromised arm. When your vest arrives,

immediately pack it with your wallet, cell phone, keys, pocket calendar, notebook, this book, medical folder, envelope for storing receipts and lab reports, water bottle, and any snacks you want to carry to prevent nausea. You may also want to include a paperback book for all the waiting time you'll likely be experiencing.

☐ A **prosthesis** (breast form) is one item you may want to wait to purchase. Most surgeons recommend you wait at least one month after surgery to wear a prosthesis, and it's extremely difficult to be properly fitted for a prosthesis until after your surgery. More guidelines can be found on p. 201.

☐ If you're planning a swimming vacation anytime soon, see p. 156 for sources of mastectomy **swimsuits**.

☐ You can get a **medical ID alert bracelet** (to notify medical staff not to draw blood or take blood pressure in your at-risk-for-lymphedema arm) at *www.CreativeMedicalID.com/womens_medical_ bracelets?b=1.* Women report varying success with using these; hospital staff members don't always pay attention.

☐ **Electric razor.** If you're at risk for lymphedema, you might want to switch from a safety razor (where it's easier to nick yourself) to an electric razor. But you can hold off on this purchase, because you might lose all your hair, including underarm hair, during

	chemotherapy.
☐	Consider purchasing a **grabber,** with a squeeze-able handle, so that, post-surgery when bending is difficult, you can pick things up that you drop (including your clothing!). You can find grabbers at *Amazon.com* for $14.
☐	You might want to consider borrowing or renting a **recliner**; some women find it too difficult to sleep in bed the first weeks after surgery, and a recliner provides the perfect amount of support. Try to get one where the recline button is not on the lower side; it might be hard for you to bend down and reach it post-surgery. Rent-A-Center (*www.RentACenter.com*) is a national chain where you can rent recliners for just $7 per week.
☐	Some women find that the surgery makes them itchy, and that an inexpensive **back scratcher** is helpful.
☐	A Camelbak **hydration system** ($35 and up) will let you drink without sitting up, and fall asleep drinking from your water bottle without spilling it all over yourself. *www.Camelbak.com/Sports-Recreation/ Packs.aspx*
☐	Some women recommend investing in an inexpensive **sound machine** for white noise, which will help you sleep both in the hospital and at home.

Day 6:
Family, Friends, and Support

ೞ ೠ

Important Note: Stop Aspirin. If you've been taking aspirin as an anti-inflammatory for cancer prevention or any other reason, **stop taking it today** and do not take it again until several weeks after your surgery. Aspirin (as well as all non-steroidal anti-inflammatories including **Advil, Motrin, and Aleve**) interferes with your body's ability to clot blood and is **not** recommended for patients about to undergo, or who have recently undergone, surgery. (Tylenol is ok to continue.) Check with your doctor about when it's advisable to re-start aspirin. Similarly, **discontinue use of ginger, garlic, and omega-3 supplements** (all of which have anticoagulant effects similar to aspirin) starting today.

Buying my nine-year-old a goldfish the day before the surgery turned out to be the single smartest thing I did, because it totally distracted her. Also it cost under a dollar. Not counting the tank, the purifier, the food, the pebbles, and the glow-in-the-dark seaweed so that the poor lonely fishie would have a nightlight, of course.

Telling Family

Telling family and friends you have cancer can be one of the hardest things you'll ever do. Here's how to approach it:

- Be honest with your children about your breast cancer: There's almost no way to keep something like this a secret, and you'll do better by leveling with them from the beginning.

- Tell your children about your breast cancer in an age-appropriate way.

- Young children may worry that your cancer is contagious, or that they are somehow to blame. Tell them: "The doctor said that nobody did anything that made me get breast cancer. And nobody can catch it from me."

- Encourage older children to maintain their normal schedule of activities despite your diagnosis; a semblance of normalcy in their lives will help them to cope. Be particularly diligent about ensuring that the children's routines are as unchanged as possible.

- Assure your kids that years ago people died from cancer because treatment wasn't effective, but now most people survive cancer. (It can be helpful to reel off a list of friends and family members whom the children know who have suffered with, and survived, breast cancer.)

- Be sure to discuss the situation with your children's teachers and guidance counselor, so that they can be alert to problems at school, and sensitive to mood swings, unfinished homework, and absences.

- Consider scheduling a field trip to the hospital with your children before your surgery, so they can have a mental image of where you'll be. Seeing where you'll be when you're away will go a long way towards alleviating kids' worries. Point out the 'fun' parts of the hospital—the elevators, the vending machines, the cafeteria, the gift shop.

- Ask your hospital if they offer books or 'goody bags' to children of breast cancer patients; many do, including toys and educational material.

- Be sure to schedule private time on a regular basis with your partner throughout the breast cancer journey. Having a regular 'date night' even if you're only able to go for a short walk or get an ice cream cone will help to normalize your experience and provide needed (and regular) emotional support.

- Likewise, make regular 'dates' with your children, so that they feel they have a regular slot of your time during a period when they might otherwise tend to fall through the cracks.

- If your children would benefit from a support group geared to kids whose parents have cancer, *www. ChildrensTreeHouseFdn.org/support.html* has listings.

(But keep in mind that support groups for children can be depressing and aren't for everyone.)

- The website *ParentingWithCancer.com* offers articles and extremely helpful advice.

Telling Friends

This is the time to reach out to friends, both local (who can be of practical assistance in helping you navigate the next few months) and long-distance (who can provide emotional support and long-distance nurturing.)

- Make a list of your friends (including email addresses and phone numbers) so you can stay in touch easily.

- Consider sending everyone a 'form letter' email to apprise them of your medical situation. It may be easier to tell everyone at once than to start telling individuals one by one. Avoid relying on Facebook updates, since they are now seen by only about 15% of your Facebook friends.

- The more open you are about your diagnosis and situation, the easier it will be for friends to reach out to you and help you, and the less awkward everyone will find it.

- Be aware that some friends will be tremendously supportive and others (sometimes even close friends) will disappear. Some people find it difficult to deal with illness, and while they may *want* to be there for you, they just can't.

- Be aware that while some friends will know what to say, others will ask insensitive questions or make wildly inappropriate comments. Hard as it may be, just shrug it off; this has more to do with *them* than with *you*.

- While it can be extremely helpful to engage the support of friends, it's important to set expectations so that you get the kind of support you need. Many people are uncomfortable with illness, in particular a life-threatening situation such as cancer, but if you're clear about what you expect, you'll have better luck getting the kind of reaction you need from your friends. Be explicit: "I'm planning to get through this with a positive attitude, so please *don't* put on a sad puppy dog face and ask me how I feel, but please *do* invite me out for coffee and to take walks."

- Be clear about your needs: Tell friends how ("Please *don't* phone me, but please do stay in touch by email") and how often ("I find more than two or three visitors a day tiring") you'd like to be contacted. Be sure to tell your partner how many, and which friends you'd like to see while in the hospital.

Dealing with People's Comments

You might find that some friends and acquaintances say comforting, lovely things to you, and others make comments that are just plain stupid. Here are some things people might say, and some responses you could make:

- "I've heard you have cancer." If you want to discuss this, you can say something like, "Thanks for bringing it up—I've been meaning to talk to you about this". But if you *don't* want to discuss this, feel free to say, "Thanks for your concern—but I'd rather not discuss my health issues right now."

- "How *are* you?!" (said in a my-puppy-just-died voice). Depending on your relationship with the person, you can say something like, "I'm feeling like crap right now, actually; want to babysit my kids for a few hours so I can nap?" or "I'm doing just fine; how are *you*?"

- "My neighbor cured her cancer with—" (fill in the blank—shark oil, vitamin therapy, bee pollen, you name it, it's been tried.) Something like, "I'll talk to my oncologist about that—thanks!" is usually the fastest way out of this conversation.

Fill-in: People to Help

People to Help		
Help Needed	Day Needed & Time	Name of Friend
Food		
Childcare		
House		
Transportation		
Shopping		
Laundry		
Other		

Finding Support

- Studies show that cancer survivors who participate in support group meetings live longer than those who don't. (The most striking study at Stanford University showed that advanced breast cancer patients who attended a two-hour support group every week lived *twice* as long as those who did not attend.) So get out there and find a group with which to hang.

- But be careful: Some cancer survivor support groups turn into depressing, sob-story evenings. If you've inadvertently stumbled onto that sort of support group, thank them nicely and find another group. What you want is a group of inspired, energetic survivors who will help your spirits stay strong, not a pity party.

- Two worthwhile online forums you might want to consider are:

  o *community.breastcancer.org*

  o Breast Cancer Social Media Tweet Chat, Monday nights at 9pm ET, on Twitter; follow *@BCSMComm, bcsm.info*

- One additional word on online lists and forums: While it's wonderful to be able to just ask people questions, online forums can be both helpful and scary. Sometimes the participants unknowingly disseminate misinformation (so always check with your doctor if you don't understand something, or if something you read contradicts something your doctor has told you) and sometimes reading about medical conditions which you might never have to experience can be more harmful than helpful. So tread carefully.

One option some women employ is to have their spouse or partner peruse the online forums for useful information, while avoiding reading it themselves.

Fill-in: Support Group

Here are some questions to ask when deciding on a support group:

Support Group	
Name of group	
When does it meet?	
Where does it meet?	
Is this group for breast cancer survivors in particular?	
How many people participate in this group?	
It is for patients only, or partners too?	
Is it only for people currently in treatment, or also for survivors?	

Is it usually a pretty upbeat crowd, or does it tend to get depressing?	

Coordinating Support

- Put together a community for support, or have your partner or a friend put a group together for you. Women who are active in a church or synagogue may find that the logical place to base their community; others may find that a support group of work friends is most helpful.

- There are many online sites that can assist communities in organizing play dates, carpools, and food; they also include message boards where friends can post greetings. These include:

  o *www.CaringBridge.org*

  o *www.LotsaHelpingHands.com*

  o *www.TakeThemAMeal.com*

  o *www.MealTrain.com*

- Provide friends (perhaps via an online forum so you can coordinate tasks more easily) with lists of:

o Housekeeping chores ("Laundry baskets are in the laundry room and washer/dryer instructions are taped to the wall.")

o Grocery shopping and meal needs ("We keep a shopping list on the refrigerator.")

o Carpooling requests ("The boys need rides home from soccer practice on Tuesdays and Thursdays.")

o Food and lifestyle preferences ("Jason is allergic to peanuts and Maggie hates tomatoes; everyone likes noodle casseroles with cheese (but no tuna!), lasagna-type dishes with or without vegetables, and meat loaf.")

o What your family prefers as takeout and on play dates: "Everyone loves pizza (with mushrooms) and fried chicken; the kids always enjoy macaroni and cheese, pita pizzas, spaghetti with tomato sauce."

• If you're changing your diet because of your diagnosis (see p. 81) be sure to create a comprehensive list of what you do and don't eat, so that friends who want to cook for you are able to accommodate your requirements. This can be as simple as a short description. Here's what we sent out upon my diagnosis to friends who asked:

> *Some of you have asked about Fern's food restrictions. We're not expecting anyone to spend the time in the kitchen messing with vegan food, which tends to be*

more time-consuming to prepare, but several of you have asked for details, so I'm posting the list of do's and don'ts here for those adventurous enough to want to try—thanks for everyone who's offered! (And the rest of us are happy eating whatever people cook for us.)

Fern's Modified Vegan Diet

- *Mostly vegan (no meat, no chicken, no eggs, no dairy.) Fish is ok.*

- *No sugars—no sugar, no honey, no maple syrup, no artificial sweeteners, no anything sweet.*

- *No white anything—no white rice, no white pasta, no white bread. (Whole wheat/whole grain/brown rice are all ok.)*

- *No soup mixes, no chemicals, no packaged products of any sort*

- *No potatoes. (All other vegetables are ok, including sweet potatoes.)*

- *Minimal fruit.*

- *Beans, lentils, etc, are ok. Seaweed is ok. Olive & sesame oils are ok. Brown rice sushi is great! Any herb or spice is ok.*

Hope this helps, and thanks to all of you who've offered to help cook, it's really appreciated.

Fill-in: Information for Helpers

You can make it easier for those who want to help you out with a meal or shopping by providing them with the information and tips below.

Information for Helpers	
Name	
Address	
Phone	
Email	
# people to cook for	# Adults_____ # Children_____
Best time to deliver meals	
Special instructions for dropping off food or gaining entry to home	
Favorite meals	

Least favorite meals	
Favorite takeout	
Food allergies	
Special instructions	
Groceries needed	
Other errands needed (library books, post-office runs, etc.)	
Best time to visit	

Checklist: Helper Etiquette

✓	Helper Etiquette
☐	Unless invited, plan to drop off meals without staying to visit.
☐	Arrive within the suggested time window.
☐	Bring enough food so that there'll be leftovers, particularly if the leftovers can be frozen for later use.
☐	Remember extras like beverages, condiments, and dessert.
☐	Consider including a special treat for young children to help them through this difficult time.
☐	If you're paying to have something delivered to the family, be sure you've covered the cost of tip and tax, and that you've specified what delivery time is optimal.
☐	If possible, deliver your meal in a disposable container so the family doesn't need to spend time scrubbing and returning serving dishes.
☐	Include clear preparation instructions, e.g., "Bake for 1 hour at 350 degrees" or "Does not need refrigeration."
☐	Consider including a note or a card. Definitely include

	your name so they know who it's from.
☐	Ask if you can drop off any groceries or supplies while you're delivering food.
☐	If you're looking for an appropriate gift for a friend in treatment, PlanetCancer offers tongue-in-cheek T-shirts and bumper-stickers, (including "I had cancer and all I got was this T-shirt" and "Don't like my driving? Tough—I had cancer") at *www.cafepress.com/planetcancer*.

Tracking Help and Things Borrowed

Later on, you'll probably want to know which friends helped out. Be sure you keep track as you go along: Use the handy tracking form in the appendix on p. 297, and ask your partner and children to write it down whenever anyone drops by or helps out.

Similarly, use the form on p. 295 to track books, DVDs, and other items friends have loaned you.

Day 7:
Planning Your Schedule

❦

Experiences with surgery and treatment vary, but most women find that they suffer from energy depletion at the very least.

Because of that, and because for most women treatment goes on for several months, one of the most important things you can do in preparation for treatment is organize your schedule.

If your family life doesn't fall apart despite your appointments and side-effects, and if you're able to continue working because you've scheduled your time and energy effectively, you'll feel much better about the whole experience, and it will be less overwhelming, not only for you, but for everyone around you. Here's how to start:

Checklist: Scheduling

✓	Scheduling
☐	If you don't already have one, buy *one* daily planner

☐	to use both for work and personal life. (Using more than one will just confuse an already fraught situation.)
☐	Sit down with the calendar, and plan out the long-standing commitments—events and parties, major obligations, outside (school, work, etc) commitments, work travel, and major project deadlines. Be realistic about what you can expect to accomplish, and be prepared to skip the items that aren't truly important—you won't be able to do everything during treatment, and expecting too much of yourself will just make you stressed.
☐	Take everything *off* the calendar that will interfere with your treatment, such as optional out-of-town trips and vacations that will interrupt your chemotherapy or radiation schedule.
☐	Schedule babysitters, housecleaning, errands, and driving arrangements.
☐	Compile the list of things that need to be done every month. Don't forget items like bill-paying, which can otherwise slip through the cracks.
☐	Compile the list of things that should be done once a year, like check the furnace, or send flowers to your mother for her birthday.

☐	Call now and make all the appointments that you know you'll need for the coming year (and get as many of them out of the way as possible before your treatment begins): Dentist, doctor, and eye appointments for all family members; and veterinarian appointments if you have a pet. By scheduling them well in advance, you can book them back-to-back, thus making fewer trips.
☐	Tap your community of friends who've offered to be available for you (see p. 115). Remind people of what help you will need, and when.
☐	Create a master to-do list of all the business and personal things you need to do. Before you schedule them on your calendar, *cut out any that are unnecessary.* This is not the year to attempt to clean out your basement or write a new book. Focus on essentials.
☐	Make a chart for your children (and partner) with age-appropriate household tasks they can help with—shopping errands, quick dinner preparation, running a load of wash. Your energy will be depleted, but you can keep your home and family life running on track if everyone pitches in to the best of his abilities.
☐	Create a 'bare minimum' list of essential chores that must be done each week: dinner, dishes, laundry, carpooling children, etc. As long as someone gets to these items, the house won't fall apart. Also, insist

	that someone be in charge of tidying and generally neatening the house every evening, so that you feel calm and organized (whether or not the closets are clean!) Be prepared to let certain tasks go: This is not the year your house will win any cleanliness awards—and that's ok.
☐	Type up your family schedule and post it inside your front door and in several prominent places throughout the house to help prevent things from falling through the cracks.
☐	Remember to schedule quality time with your spouse and children. Especially during the months of treatments, this will be important—for both you and them. Even if you're not up for anything strenuous, you can join them on a coffee date or a walk through the park.
☐	Block out times for exercise. Chemotherapy patients vary in how energetic they are and how much they can do, so if you're energetic, keep up your regular gym workouts; if you're less energetic, at least make the time to get out there and walk, every day if possible. (This will make a huge difference in how you feel, and for many people, it also helps with nausea and side-effects.)
☐	Organize a childcare plan for the days of and immediately following your surgery. (Even if you have a partner, it's better to make an independent plan for

	the kids if possible; you'll want your partner to be at your bedside at least part of the time.) If your children are younger, then the easiest solution might be to have a close friend come in to care for them. If they're older, they might prefer to go to friends' for an overnight or two.
☐	If you have pets, be sure you've asked someone to feed/water/walk them.
☐	If you'll need chemotherapy, organize a plan for your children on the days you'll be having treatment: If the treatments take longer than you anticipate, you won't have the additional worry of untended children standing forlornly at your locked door; and even if you're home on schedule, you'll have a few extra hours to rest up before having to deal with the commotion of normal family life. A regularly-scheduled play date or activity the afternoon of your chemotherapy treatments can be a lifesaver, and could be something your child will look forward to as well.
☐	You might want to schedule a hair appointment for sometime before your surgery, since you probably won't be able to shampoo your own hair for several weeks (because it will be difficult to raise your hands above your head post-surgery)
☐	Since you won't be able to lift anything for a while, stock up on any heavy items that you need on a

	regular basis (laundry detergent, dog food, bottled water).
☐	Rent a few movies that you particularly want to see, so you have something to look forward to when you come home from the hospital. If you rent family movies, your whole gang can enjoy watching with you.
☐	Make sure that your surgeon, the hospital, and the insurance company all have your cell phone number: If they need to reach you pre-operation, it's helpful if they don't have to wait to hear back from you until you hear the messages on your home machine. If you're reluctant to be 'on call' for everyone, give out the cell phone number of your partner or a friend.
☐	Type up multiple copies of your current medications list, so that you can give them to each doctor and member of the hospital staff that needs it.
☐	Be sure that you and your partner both have the phone number of your closest-to-home pharmacy on your cell phones.
☐	While you're organizing, type up a list of your user names and passwords for all the websites you use frequently, particularly anything of a financial ilk. The stress and trauma of surgery (and then chemotherapy) may flush your brain of useful information, and if you're passing off some of the

	responsibilities to a partner or friend, having that information written down somewhere might alleviate some of the stress. Just be sure to keep it in a secure place.
☐	Organize healthy snacks for your hospital stay; if you're on a restricted diet or cancer diet, organize the actual meals (with instructions for your partner or a friend on what to bring and when, and how to prepare it if there's preparation necessary.)
☐	Use the log in the appendix on p. 295 for tracking items you've borrowed (and items you've lent out.)
☐	Consider allocating one of your credit cards as your health care card, and consistently pay for all treatment-related items with that card. This makes tax returns much easier, and lets you more easily track proof of payment should questions arise.

Day 8:
Guided Visualization

ೞ ೞ

*M*any *friends suggested the apparently common tactic of employing the "your internal army is battling the cancer" imagery to fight my cancer, but in the end, I opted for something less militaristic. My 'army', honestly, seems to have been on something of a vacation for the duration; now that the invaders have breached the castle walls seems not necessarily the best time to begin galvanizing the troops for action. Basically they, like me, have been on coffee break for far too long :*)*

Guided visualization is a way to tap into the mind-body connection. People use different techniques to visualize cancer cells shrinking and retreating: Some imagine the cancer cells as small squirmy insects, running around in confusion; some imagine the cancer as shrinking bits of protoplasm, others use military imagery of retreating armies.

Checklist: Guided Visualization

Guided visualization can be effective both for surgery and chemotherapy. Here are some tips on 'visualizing' yourself to optimal health:

✓	Guided Visualization
☐	At least once a day, imagine your cancer leaving your body.
☐	You might find it helpful to get a book on guided visualization and put together an audio that you can listen to regularly, telling yourself that you'll be healthy and strong.
☐	Ask your surgeon if you can bring your audio and headset into the operating room, so that you can listen to it while you're undergoing surgery. Some experts maintain that even when you are under anesthesia you can 'hear' suggestions, and that these suggestions will make your recovery much easier.
☐	Avoid using words like 'weak' and 'pain' and even 'cancer' on your tape because that just reinforces those connections in your mind; don't use negative words at all. Instead, focus on phrases like, "My body is getting stronger and feeling healthy" and "My operation has gone so well, this has been a really successful operation!"

☐	Describe how you envision getting rid of the cancer (again, without using the word 'cancer'): "Those weak, confused, shrinking cells are scurrying out of my body. I'm filled with energy and with healing light. There are red carpets throughout my body, and I'm going to walk down those red carpets with those little, weak cells and escort them out. Once the surgery escorts them out, my chemotherapy is going to sweep up after them and I'm going to feel fabulous!"
☐	Then, describe how you feel after the surgery, again remembering to keep the description positive, rather than negative: "I'm coming out of the surgery. I feel comfortable and rested. My body feels calm and peaceful. My arm feels strong and comfortable."
☐	Describe a scene that you'd like to occur about a day after surgery: "It's a day after the surgery, and I'm recovering and healing really happily. I'm feeling great! Let's go out for dinner and a walk."
☐	Describe a scene many years in the future: "I see myself with my children and grandchildren, all together and happy. I am totally cured, healed, and feeling great. I still work out every day, and I feel fantastic."
☐	You may also want to include suggestions telling your body that you'll wake up hungry, thirsty, and able to urinate and defecate easily, so that your body systems

	are galvanized to wake up easily from the anesthesia.
☐	Consider putting peaceful, lulling background music onto your audio, to further impel you to relax while listening.
☐	A personalized audio will probably prove more beneficial than a generic tape, because you can tailor it to your personal situation and concerns, but if you're not up for making your own audio, try the following resources: • Peggy Huddleston's "Prepare for Surgery, Heal Faster" ($35 for both the book and audio) at *www.HealFaster.com* • While not a guided visualization per se, Jon Kabat-Zinn's "Full Catastrophe Living: Using the Wisdom of Your Body and Mind to Face Stress, Pain and Illness" (available in both book and audio format at Amazon or at Zinn's website *MindfulnessCDs .com*) or his one-hour "The World of Relaxation" audio (used in many hospitals) available (for $12 audio download, $17 CD) at *shop.betterlisten .com/products/world-of-relaxation-a-guided-mindfulness-meditation-practice-for-healing-in-the-hospital-and-or-at-home.*
☐	Besides making an audio for your surgical experience, consider doing a similar audio for your chemotherapy treatments.

☐ Finally, if you're going to use the audio during surgery, be sure that the volume is set correctly, that the controls can't be jiggered accidentally (try a piece of scotch tape over the controls), and that there are new batteries installed so that the audio will play the entire duration of your surgery. Don't forget to ask your surgeon in advance in case there's a procedure that needs to be followed.

Day 9:
Fun and Free Resources

❦ ❧

There are dozens of free resources available for breast cancer survivors. Though it is wonderful that so many programs exist, it can be overwhelming to try to wade through the sheer volume of breast cancer offerings, particularly when you're dealing with so many other things. Rather than plunge into the overwhelming morass of options, we've included just a short list of a few of the best of the fun and free resources to look into.

- You can participate in a (free) 12-week program at many YMCAs that combines exercise, lymphedema therapy, and other cancer-related education. *www.Livestrong.org/What-We-Do/Our-Actions/ Programs-Partnerships/LIVESTRONG-at-the-YMCA*

- If the Livestrong program isn't available in your location, ask whether there are any other cancer-survivor programs available; many YMCAs run shorter versions, also at no charge. Some YMCAs also offer the Breast Cancer Survivor's 12-week "Pink Program" Fitness Plan; ask your local Y.

- You can get (free) support via mail, including greeting cards and the occasional gift, from Chemo Angels at *www.ChemoAngels.net*. Cancer survivors are assigned two 'angels' who keep in touch by mail (and sometimes email).

- Look Good, Feel Better (*LookGoodFeelBetter.org*) offers free two-hour workshops by cosmeticians to teach you how to look better (through judicious use of makeup and wigs) while undergoing chemotherapy and cancer treatment. Workshops also include a lovely batch of free makeup supplies for each participant.

- Local chapters of the American Cancer Society sometimes offer free wigs. You can check directly with them to see if free wigs are offered in your geographic area. *www.Cancer.org*

- You can get a beautiful complimentary headscarf (along with a hand-written card with well-wishes) from *www.GoodWishesScarves.org*.

- You can get free housecleaning. Maid services across the US offer four free cleanings (one per month for four months total) *www.CleaningForAReason.org/ page/contact_us*

- If you're on the east coast and you are under age 40, the Tiger Lily Foundation (*www.TigerLilyFoundation .org*) provides eight free meal deliveries. They also provide free 'buddy bags' with cosmetic gifts and scarves.

- Gods Love We Deliver also provides free meals to cancer patients. *www.GLWD.org/clients/become.jsp*

- If it is necessary or beneficial for you to travel for your treatment, be aware that the American Cancer Society offers over 30 'Hope Lodges' around the country where you (and your family) can stay temporarily at no charge. Call the American Cancer Society at (800) 227-2345 for more details. The National Association of Hospital Hospitality Houses also provides free accommodations to those seeking medical treatment outside their hometown: *www.NAHHH.org* or (800) 542-9730.

- You can get free local transportation to treatment by calling the American Cancer Society and asking about their Road to Recovery program, (800) 227-2345. If you need long-distance transport, you can get a free ride on a corporate jet by contacting the Corporate Angel Network at *www.CorpAngelNetwork.org* or (866) 328-1313.

- You can get a free pair of cotton prostheses, knitted by volunteers. E-mail *info@TheKnittingExperience.com*.

- If you're in North Carolina you can get a free post-surgery camisole (and tote bag) made by volunteers. Contact Glennie Daniels at *Glennie_Daniels@ NCSU.edu*.

- If you're in Westchester County, New York, you can get free meals from local restaurants, free house cleaning, and free wash-and-fold laundry services from *www. CommunityCares.org*.

- Be aware that many hospitals offer a cancer center, often with free information and other free resources. Ask your doctors if there is such a center in your area.

- For free spa and free vacation opportunities, see p. 158.

Day 10:
Working Through Breast
Cancer

CƷ ঠC

If you're unemployed or self-employed, you may face worries about surviving financially or getting it all done while you go through treatment; if you're employed in a 'regular' job, you may be concerned about how you'll work through treatment. Here are some suggestions:

Telling Co-Workers

- If you're having a lumpectomy and radiation (rather than a mastectomy and chemotherapy), you might be able to conceal your treatment from your office. But, you'll also be depriving yourself of the support that you might receive from bosses and coworkers. And you might want that understanding, particularly if your job involves something that will be particularly difficult— such as lots of long-distance travel that might interfere with your treatment schedule. If you're going through chemotherapy, there's probably no good way to keep it from your co-workers, even if that's your preference.

- Rather than sharing details with the entire office, you could decide to tell just your immediate supervisor, so that your work responsibilities are appropriately tailored to your situation, without having 'everyone' know.

- However, most women find that, unless you tell no one, word gets out, so it might be better to control how and when you tell coworkers.

- The easiest way to spread the word might be via group email (unless that's clearly not your work culture.)

Setting Expectations

- As with telling friends, it's best to set expectations: Telling coworkers "I'm planning to truck on as if there's nothing happening, so please don't keep asking me how I'm feeling," or "It would be helpful for me if you checked in by email on chemotherapy weeks to see if I need help with this project," will help your coworkers feel like they're giving you what you need, and will help you get the support you need while not being smothered in undesirable ways.

- You'll probably also want to be frank with co-workers about likely treatment side-effects (hair loss, fatigue, etc.) so that they're prepared for the changes.

- Since you can't really know in advance how you're going to respond to treatment, it's wise not to make promises about whether you'll be meeting your work responsibilities. Simply say that it's going to be a challenging time, and you're going to do the best you can.

- If there are specific things coworkers can help with, such as pitching in to cover you for the extended travel that your chemotherapy schedule will prohibit, be forthright about asking for this help.

- If you'd prefer to take time off during treatment, and can afford to do so, sit down with your boss to see the best way to handle your responsibilities while you're away.

- If you're hoping to take time off from work, you might also want to sit down with human resources and see if there are provisions for disability pay, and whether that is an option. (The state in which you live may also provide some sort of short-term disability; inquire.)

Other Tips on Working Through Treatment

- If you plan to work through treatment, think about whether there are side-effects that will impede your ability to do so, and how you can deal with these. For example, if you currently do a lot of work that exposes you daily to many people (and their germs) think about whether there's a way to offload those responsibilities, or to protect yourself while still doing your job.

- If you find yourself developing 'chemo brain' and are having difficulty concentrating or remembering things you need to, be sure you are meticulous about keeping your calendar and work log organized so that you can track:

  o Meetings
  o Commitments
  o Conversations
  o Decisions
  o Deadlines
  o Responsibilities

- Organize your work must-do's. If it's not absolutely essential for the next few months, take it off the list. Then, block out time for work based on your anticipated treatment schedule. (For example, I scheduled my treatments for Tuesdays, so I front-loaded all my clients and other critical work on Sundays and Mondays, and then was able to take off every Tuesday, and work at a more relaxed pace later in the week.)

- If working at the office will prove difficult, consider whether working from home for the duration of your treatment might be a feasible option, and how you can present it to your boss.

- If you own your own business, you might choose to cut back on your hours during treatment; alternatively, you could hire temporary help to fill in the gaps, or just work around your treatment schedule.

Legalities

- If your company employs more than 50 people, and you're a full time employee who's worked there for more than a year, you're covered by the federal Family and Medical Leave Act, which allows you to take 12 weeks of unpaid time from work without losing benefits or your position.

- If you're unemployed at the time of your diagnosis, keep in mind that you don't need to tell prospective employers about your medical condition, and it is illegal for them to ask. (However, you'll probably need to tell prospective employers about accommodations you'll need due to your treatment.)

If You Can't Work

Social Security can provide benefits (both social security disability and supplemental security income) to breast cancer patients.

- You may qualify for a *compassionate allowance* if you've been diagnosed as Stage IV; you'll need to provide a pathology and operative report. You won't receive benefits for at least five months after the paperwork is filed. *www.ssa.gov/compassionate allowances*

- You may qualify for *disability benefits* depending on your diagnosis, including if you have inflammatory carcinoma, distant metastases, metastases to ten or more axillary nodes, or recurrent carcinoma. *www.ssa.gov/disability/disability_starter_kits_adult_ eng.htm*

  You may qualify for a *medical-vocational allowance* if your cancer is not as advanced as the disability listing requires, but you still have lessened functional capacity to work, including inability to lift and carry items, and shortened length of time you are able to stand, sit, and walk. If you're told you can only do sedentary work, and are over age 50, you may have a good chance of getting benefits via the medical-vocational allowance.

- You can call the Social Security Administration at (800) 772-1213 for more information, see their website at *www.ssa.gov*, or visit your local Social Security office; you can locate the nearest office using the website: *www.ssa.gov/locator*.

The vast majority of women find that they are able to work, at least to some extent, through treatment, so don't be discouraged.

Day 11:
Planning Your End-of-Treatment Vacation

౮౩ ౩౦

One of the best things you can do, pre-surgery, is to plan the vacation you're going to take once your treatment is over. A planned vacation will give you something to look forward to, take your mind off your treatment, and thanks to a handful of wonderful organizations, can be almost or entirely free of charge for breast cancer survivors. Here are some things to consider in your planning:

Checklist:
Planning Your End-of-Treatment Vacation

✓	Planning Your End-of-Treatment
☐	Remember to plan your vacation to limit sun exposure; certain chemotherapy drugs increase your risk of sunburn. And irradiated skin is more sensitive to sunburn, especially in the first year after

	treatment.
☐	Remember to guard your (bald) head from the sun with a hat or scarf, and to wear a high-neck bathing suit to protect your radiation-sensitive spots.
☐	Both chemotherapy and radiation can benefit from (mild) exercise; if you're swimming for exercise, remember to shower off the chlorine which can irritate already-sensitive post-radiation skin. (If you're currently undergoing chemotherapy and your white counts are low, or you're in the midst of radiation, your doctor may recommend that you avoid swimming entirely.)
☐	Don't alter your radiation or chemotherapy schedule to accommodate a vacation; better to change your vacation plans to accommodate your treatments. Or ask about setting up a treatment in another location if necessary.
☐	In packing for vacation, bring along all your medications and your medical records, in case a medical appointment proves necessary.
☐	If there'll be swimming opportunities, you may want to invest in a mastectomy swimsuit that can be worn with a breast form. (See details on breast forms appropriate for swimming on p. 203, or just use a net "poof", or "loofah"—the kind used for shower exfoliation—which will dry quickly.) The following

major retailers all offer mastectomy swimsuits, as do many other physical and online retailers.

- *www.LandsEnd.com/ix/swimwear-swimsuits/ Swim/Women/D-DD-DDD/mastectomy-suits/ index.html?tab=6&store=le &catNumbers=644~645~2733~3118 &visible=1~2~1~1~1*
- *www.Sears.com/health-wellness-mastectomy/ c-1024548*
- *shop.Nordstrom.com/c/prosthesis-program*
- *www.Amoena.com/us/Products/Swimwear/2012*
- *www.Jodee.com/mastectomyswimwear.jsp? cid=BT*
- *www.WomansPersonalHealth.com/swimwear/ mastectomy-swimsuits-2011-collection*

☐ If you'll be on Tamoxifen at the time of your vacation, ask your doctor about taking low-dose aspirin before (and while) you fly; aspirin is a blood-thinner, and may counteract the possibility of a Tamoxifen-induced blood clot.

☐ Be sure to notify your hosts of any relevant physical limitations. For example, your neuropathy may mean you'll be happiest on the ground floor so you don't have to stumble up stairs, or that you'll find it too challenging to bike or climb ropes.

☐ If you're worried that your cancer treatment is going

to somehow trigger alarms from the airport's Transportation Security Administration officials (because of your infusion port, or if you're sporting lymphedema wraps or other unusual accoutrements) you can contact the TSA directly to ask how to handle your situation: Call (866) 289-9673 or email *TSA-ContactCenter@dhs.gov*.

Free Vacations

There are several free or extremely low-cost retreats, camps, and vacations open only to breast cancer patient and survivors. Here is a partial listing; check with the organizations for more details:

- Betty J. Borry Breast Cancer Retreats—New England. These three-day adventure-based retreats take place in various retreat centers and outdoor facilities in New England several times each year. Some of them occur at Appalachian Mountain Club cabins. $200 usually includes accommodations (sometimes in bunk rooms with shared baths, for other retreats in more upscale housing), all meals, hiking/ropes/skiing and programming; limited to about 20 participants. *BJBBreastCancerRetreats.org*

- Bluebird Cancer Retreats—Michigan. These frequent three-day retreats, geared to both solo survivors and couples (survivor and partner), take place on the shores of Lake Michigan and include holistic therapies and reflection time. $100 per person includes accommodations, meals and all activities.   *www.BluebirdMI.org/pg/Retreats*

- Bluebonnet Retreat—Texas. Three-day retreat focused on arts and crafts, physical activities, sharing/caring time, and cancer education, at the Star Brand Ranch, an 8,000-acre ranch with a fitness center, fishing, hiking, hayrides, tennis, ping pong, and more. Free. *www.TexasHealth.org/body.cfm?id=2072*

- Bravehearts—New York.   Bravehearts offers several weekends, geared to different activities (sailing, ropes course and horseback riding, mind/body focus) in upstate New York retreat centers. $100 includes everything. *BraveHeartsCamp.org/camps.html*

- The Breast Cancer Recovery Foundation offers a variety of four-day wellness retreats on Madeline Island, Wisconsin. $400 includes accommodations, meals, and all activities; scholarships are available.   *www.BCRecovery.org/pages/Retreats.php*

- You can camp for free in the Poconos, NY at Camp Can-Doo. *www.MtPoconoCampground.com*

- Camp Good Days—New York.   Camp Good Days provides women's wellness camping weekends (focusing on therapeutic massage, yoga, meditation, reiki, manicures, and recreational activities) and women's adventure programs (with fishing, boating, swimming, rock climbing, and ropes courses.) On the shores of Keuka Lake in Yates County, New York. *www.CampGoodDays.org*

- Camp Living Springs—Florida. Camp Living Springs offers a three-day fall retreat in the 100-acre rustic wooded property in Ellenton, Florida. Free. *www. MortonPlant.com/body.cfm?id=1438*

- Camp Mak-a-Dream—Montana. Camp Mak-a-Dream offers four and five-day retreats with educational workshops, recreation, entertainment, art projects, and off-campus excursions. Includes large bunkroom accommodations and buffet style food; the lodge includes an art studio, health center, swimming pool, hot tub, ropes course, climbing wall, and hiking trails. Free. *www.CampDream.org*

- Casting for Recovery (PO Box 1123, Manchester, Vermont, 05254 (888) 553-3500) offers free, three-day fly fishing weekends for breast cancer survivors in many locations across the US. Selection is by lottery, and applicants who are shut out will be first on the waitlist for the next available program. *CastingFor Recovery.org*.

- Creative Healing Connections—New York. Creative Healing Connections at Great Camp Sagamore in the Adirondack Mountains of upstate New York offers three-day arts and healing retreats with storytelling, songwriting, dreamwork, and visual arts. *www. CreativeHealingConnections.org/retreats*

- First Descents—various locations. First Descents offers free week-long adventure experiences (whitewater kayaking, rock climbing, surfing) for cancer survivors under age 39. *FirstDescents.org*

- Harmony Hill—Washington. Harmony Hill offers three-day retreats (some for survivors, others for survivors and partners) focusing on stress reduction, guided imagery, movement, and massage. Food, lodging, and program at no charge. *www.HarmonyHill.org/node/26*

- Healing Odyssey offers three-day weekend ropes courses in Santa Barbara, California for cancer survivors. Courses are highly-subsidized ($299 includes all accommodations, meals, and the course itself, and full financial aid is available for those who will have difficulty paying.) *www.HealingOdyssey.org*

- Little Pink Houses of Hope—North and South Carolina. Little Pink Houses of Hope offers free week-long beach houses (including lodging, meals, and all activities) in resort areas of North and South Carolina beaches. Each family is housed in their own beach house, with common meals and programming (kayaking, hang gliding, paddle boarding, golf, jewelry making, massage, fishing, sailing, concerts) for the group. *LittlePinkHousesofHope.org*

- Odyssey offers free low-stress adventure vacations in the UK; you need to be recommended by your doctor or hospital for this program. *www.Odyssey.org.uk*

- Reeling and Healing—midwest. Reeling & Healing Fly Fishing Retreats are 3-day retreats in the midwest for those with no prior fly fishing experience. $25 includes accommodations, meals, and equipment, in various midwest locations. *ReelingandHealingMidwest.org/ programs.php*

- Sail4Cancer offers free British sailing events and vacations. See the schedule at *www.Sail4Cancer.org.*

- Stowe Weekend of Hope—Stowe, Vermont. Stowe Weekend of Hope offers free bed and breakfast accommodations (plus free programs) in the resort town of Stowe, Vermont during their cancer education weekend each spring. *StoweHope.org*

- Women Beyond Cancer—location varies. Women Beyond Cancer offers three-day retreats in South Carolina (horseback riding), Utah (adventure), Maine (yoga/nutrition), and Zion National Park (adventure). Free. *WomenBeyondCancer.org/retreats.html*

Day 12:
Preparing for Surgery

❦ ❧

There are some things you can do to prepare for surgery (and your return from the hospital) that will make your entire experience less stressful.

Checklist: Preparing for Surgery

✓	Preparing for Surgery
☐	To prevent theft, remove your wedding ring and any other jewelry when you pack for the hospital. (Be sure to tell your partner or friend *where* you're putting your wedding ring so that you can easily find it afterwards.)
☐	Similarly, if you have an expensive cell phone or computer, leave it at home to avoid theft, and buy an inexpensive disposable cell phone for your hospital stay.
☐	Plan to have someone drive you home after your hospital stay. (You may also need to arrange for

	someone to help you out at home for a few days post-surgery.)
☐	Don't forget to pack suitcases for your children, if they'll be going elsewhere.
☐	You might want to pack a small bag for your partner if he'll be staying in the hospital with you, including: • Sleepwear • Change of clothing • Contact lens solution, toothbrush, etc. • An iTunes gift card for movies or music, or a paperback he'll enjoy • Quarters for the vending machines • Healthy snacks • Take-out menus for emergency food runs for the kids at home
☐	Consider leaving love notes and small gifts for each of your children for the time that you'll be in the hospital—just to remind them that you love them, and that even when things are rough, you're thinking of them.
☐	Before you leave for the hospital, set up your bed and nightstand, so that when you arrive home, you're able to reach everything easily. You'll need a lot of pillows (including extra pillows for under your back and legs, and maybe for under your arms as well.) Within arm's reach on your nightstand you'll probably want your

	phone, your medication, tissues, bottled water, your remote control, and a book or iPod. In the bathroom, you'll want a measuring cup in which to empty your drain, and pen or pencil to record the quantities.
☐	Empty your shampoo, conditioner, and body soap into trial sized bottles (which you can get at any drugstore). The larger bottles might be too heavy for you to comfortably lift, post-surgery.
☐	Place any items you'll need for showering (shampoo, conditioner, soap) in an accessible location, or perhaps hanging from a mesh bag; it will be difficult for you to reach overhead, and similarly difficult for you to bend down, post-surgery.
☐	Pull out some light plastic cups to drink from if you usually use (heavy) mugs.
☐	Move your most commonly-used kitchen items to lower shelves pre-surgery, so that you won't have to lift your arms to reach things.
☐	Unless you have young children, transfer your medication into *non* child-proof cap bottles, because you will find opening child-proof medicine caps particularly challenging post-surgery.
☐	If you'll be having chemotherapy, toss your old cosmetic products (which can cause infection) and replace with new cosmetics.

Checklist: Packing for the Hospital

✓	Packing for the Hospital
☐	Toiletries—toothbrush, toothpaste, contact lens solution and case, spare glasses, comb, etc.
☐	Healthy snacks and/or entire meals, if you're determined to stick to a particular diet
☐	Recharger for your cell phone and an inexpensive or throw-away cell phone
☐	Photos of family members, in small frames. Not only will the family photos make you feel good when you look at them, but the nursing staff find people in some sort of context easier to relate to (and people with photos of kids also provide an easy conversation topic) so this might actually improve your care.
☐	An eye mask and earplugs if you're sensitive to light and sound; hospitals are noisy places.
☐	An (inexpensive) way to listen to music.
☐	Oversized clothing; some women find that they have a big problem with swelling, and your 'regular' size might not fit until the swelling abates. Include a comfortable post-surgery outfit in which to go home. (Be sure this has loose, easy openings, and includes a button-up shirt; it may be hard for you to get a pullover on, you might find it challenging to raise your

☐	hands in the air post-surgery.)
☐	If getting a lumpectomy, be sure to pack your sports bra.
☐	If you have long hair, pack ponies or hair bands to keep your hair out of the way in the hospital.
☐	Lip balm—hospitals are dry places.
☐	Health insurance card and details
☐	Complete medical records (just in case)
☐	A contact list of your friends and family, along with phone numbers, so you can reach people from the hospital.
☐	A robe to wear over your hospital gown in case of visitors
☐	Underwear, non-skid slip-on slippers, warm socks (because hospital rooms are sometimes refrigerators)
☐	This book
☐	Your guided visualization tape, headset, and spare batteries
☐	Notepad and pen for taking notes

☐	Large envelope for taking home hospital documentation
☐	A copy of the details of where your children will be while you're in the hospital (see below) in case you need to call or change things.

Fill-in:
Organizing Children For Mom's Surgery

If your children are going elsewhere while you're in the hospital, pack their suitcases carefully to be sure they have everything they'll need (including a comfort object). Include a checklist (below) both of what they need to bring/pack (homework, stuffed animal with which to sleep, change of clothes, PJs) and what they need to remember to do (cello lesson is Monday afternoon, bring ballet slippers to school, etc.) Be sure to include a few 'love notes' and maybe a small gift or two so they know you're thinking about them. All this advance preparation will help you—and them—feel less stressed on the day of the surgery. Include a small gift for their host in their suitcase.

If your children are staying with different friends, provide this list to all of them so siblings can be in touch. Remember to take a copy to the hospital, too, just in case.

Organizing Children For Mom's Surgery

Name of child			
Child's cell phone			
Name of host			
Address			
Phone			
Child's schedule	Day	Activity	Equipment needed
	Sun		
	Mon		
	Tues		
	Wed		
	Thu		
	Fri		
	Sat		

What to pack for your kids	• Toiletries • PJs • Bathrobe and slippers • Underwear, socks • Change of outfit • School backpack and books • Musical instrument or sports equipment needed for school or after-school • Love notes and small gifts • Stuffed animal • Hostess gift

Day 13:
Last-Minute Reminders

ℭℬ ℬ

Here are just a few last-minute reminders before your surgery:

Checklist: Last-Minute Reminders

✓	Last-Minute Reminders
☐	If you're having a sentinel node biopsy, remember to ask your doctor about taking Tylenol (not aspirin nor any non-steroidal anti-inflammatory, including Advil, Motrin, or Aleve, all of which impair blood clotting and therefore shouldn't be taken before surgery) to dull the pain of the shot that you'll receive, which some women claim is the most painful part of the entire operation.
☐	If you're having a mastectomy, prepare in advance a ribbon that can comfortably fasten around your neck (and that can easily get over your head) to anchor your drainage tubes while showering, or plan to borrow one of your spouse's little-used ties for this.

	(See p 103)
☐	If you're going to use a guided visualization tape during surgery (see p. 139), be sure you've informed the medical staff and that you have new batteries installed in your portable music player.
☐	Put a "Thank You Log" and a pen near your front door, so that your family can easily keep track of which friends stopped by to visit, dropped off casseroles, helped run your kids around in carpool, etc.
☐	Scatter alcohol-gel hand sanitizer dispensers or sani-wipes strategically through the house, including at the front door (along with a prominently visible sign for guests, insisting that they wash before entering.) Your immune system will be compromised, and the more you can do to prevent germs from entering your home, the healthier you will stay.
☐	Remember to get quart containers of items like milk and orange juice; immediately post-surgery, you'll find lifting gallon jugs challenging.
☐	Write notes to your kids and partner reminding them of how much you love them, and leave the notes around your house for them to find. This will reassure them during what will be a challenging emotional time.

Day 14:
Take a Mini-Vacation

ભ્ર ૯૦

Right before your surgery, take a one-day or overnight vacation.

- Take your whole family if you'll find that most relaxing and enjoyable, or just your partner if that's preferable. (Don't forget to book a babysitter well in advance if you're going solo.)

- If you can't afford or don't want an overnight in a hotel, plan an all-day outing with meal stops and activities you'll enjoy.

- Try a new art museum or gallery, go bowling, head to the new boutique you've been meaning to explore—whatever sounds like fun.

- Start by asking everyone to turn off their cell phones.

- Bring along a camera, and during the day snap pictures of your family enjoying themselves.

- Post the photos on Facebook, along with an update telling friends that you're en route to the hospital; this is likely to remind friends that your surgery is approaching, and will help ensure that your family gets the support it needs while you're in treatment.

The Post-Surgery Recovery Checklist

CZ ЯD

Your surgeon and hospital may give you post-surgery instructions, including on pain management, incision care, diet, and follow-up. In cases where our suggestions contradict the instructions you've received from your doctor or hospital, follow your doctor's directions.

In the Hospital

- The length of your surgery will be determined by exactly what is being done (lumpectomy, mastectomy, reconstruction, etc.) A 'typical' mastectomy with lymph node removal will take about four hours.

- Likewise, the length of your hospital stay will depend on your surgery (and, unfortunately, your insurance). Mastectomy patients, including those who have had expander reconstruction, generally stay overnight. If you've had flap reconstruction, the hospital stay will likely be 3-4 nights. Lumpectomy (without axillary lymph node dissection) will usually be done on an outpatient basis.

- Most women will have little pain, though you may experience numbness or pulling in the under-arm area. Pain may actually be worst a few days *post*-surgery.

- You will likely have between one and four drainage tubes (surgically attached to your chest) to remove fluid. After a week or two, once the fluid flow has decreased, the surgeon will remove the drains.

Checklist: Before You Leave the Hospital

✓	Before You Leave the Hospital
☐	Nurses may urge you to sit up (in chairs) rather than lay down (in your bed) because they believe sitting will prevent pneumonia that hospital patients are prone to. (Plus-sized women may want to request a larger chair or a wheelchair in which to sit if the chair is an uncomfortable fit.)
☐	Don't leave the hospital until you have emptied your drainage tubes while a nurse watches you—just to make sure you understand how to do it correctly.
☐	Ask the nursing staff to show you how to get in and out of bed, post-surgery, without straining your back.
☐	Have whoever is going to drive you home from the hospital bring a small pillow, to put between your surgery scar and the car's shoulder straps.

☐	Have your spouse or friend fill any necessary drugstore prescriptions in advance, so that you don't have to stop on the way home from the hospital.

Fill-in: Follow-Up Care

Before leaving the hospital, ask for instructions (preferably in writing) as to:

Follow-Up Care	
How to care for the surgical dressing	
How to care for the drains	
How to know if there's an infection	
What arm exercises to do to prevent stiffness	
When to start wearing a bra	
When to start wearing a prosthesis or breast form	

What painkiller to take	
What activities to avoid	
When to schedule a follow-up appointment	
Whether it's ok to drive post-surgery	
When to resume normal activity	
When to resume exercise	
When to resume sexual activity	
When to expect scars to be healed	
When to bathe and shower normally	
When to call the doctor or hospital	

Checklist: At Home Post-Surgery

✓	At Home Post-Surgery
☐	After a mastectomy, you should expect to be up and around in a week or two; after reconstruction with flaps, recovery is closer to six to eight weeks. (Bruising will also last up to eight weeks after reconstruction.) Be aware that you might feel pain immediately after surgery that subsides as the days go by, or you might find that you begin to feel *more* pain a few days post-surgery. As long as the pain doesn't increase severely, both of these are normal. If the pain does increase severely, call your doctor.
☐	Avoid overhead lifting and strenuous sports for at least 4-6 weeks after reconstruction, or if you've had lymph nodes removed.
☐	It's important to start exercising your arm immediately (particularly if there were many lymph nodes removed) to maximize future mobility. Your doctor or the hospital physical therapist will show you exercises to do, or see (p. 273) for suggestions.
☐	If you've had immediate reconstruction, some surgeons recommend wearing a (very tight) underwire bra, 24/7, for three to four months, starting as soon as you've had the drainage tubes removed, to provide 'encapsulation' of the implants (basically, because nothing else is supporting the implants until

☐	scar tissue forms.) Rumors that underwire bras can somehow adversely affect the implants are apparently unsubstantiated.
☐	If you've had reconstruction, call your doctor immediately if you notice skin changes, excessive swelling, lumps, or fluid leaking from the flap donor site.
☐	Navigating the shower post-surgery will be challenging. Some women report success with a shower stool and hand-held shower nozzle; others just move plastic lawn chairs into the shower.
☐	Keep your cell phone (or a loud bell) near your bed, and if you need to reach your partner or whoever is helping you out post-surgery, call or ring them rather than trying to yell to get their attention.
☐	If you're given several medications that need to be taken at different times of day, label the bottles with masking tape and write on each what time of day you need to take it: "6 am, 10 am, 2 pm"—so that you don't get confused. Some people also find a pill-organizer useful.
☐	In the weeks after surgery, sit on the opposite side of the car from where you had the surgery, so that the car's shoulder straps don't cut into your scar.
☐	Once your surgical scar begins to heal, some women

	recommend applying A&D or vitamin E; ask your doctor.
☐	You may experience all different kinds of tingling and itching pains in your arm and hand as the nerves heal; that's normal.
☐	If you've had a lumpectomy, you might feel a hard mass at the surgery site; this is usually a build-up of fluid, and is normal (but check with your doctor).
☐	Remember to send a thank you note, flowers, or candy to your medical team—the surgeon, the oncologist, any nurses who were particularly kind, receptionists who helped you out, etc.

Checklist: Drainage Care

Most women post-surgery end up with between one and four (sometimes more) fist-sized drainage bulbs attached to tubes under the chest skin near their incisions. The drains are somewhat disgusting, but they prevent blood and fluid buildup.

When you check out of the hospital your doctor will give you a measuring cup and a log sheet, and ask you to drain the fluid frequently, and keep track of how much fluid is draining. (When it's less than about 2 tablespoons in a 24-hour period, the surgeon will remove the drain.)

- If the incision site becomes red or puffy, it might be infected—call your doctor.

- If the site is sore, try a cold compress.

- You may see small clots, bits of blood, and other solid-looking bits in the drain or tube. Don't be alarmed; it's normal, and by the time the drains are removed, it's mostly clear.

- To avoid pain when the drainage tube tugs at the incision, secure the drains to your clothing. There are a few ways to do this; see p. 103 for details of your options.

Here's how to care for your drainage tubes:

✓	Drainage Care
☐	Empty your drain every four to six hours. Take out your measuring cup (if your drain doesn't have measurements showing volume) and log sheet, as well as a clean towel on which to rest the drains (to avoid putting them down on a bacteria-laden surface.)
☐	Wash your hands thoroughly.
☐	Clean the site of the incision with a Q-tip dipped in peroxide, and water (or ask your doctor what to use)
☐	Unpin or pull out the drain from your clothing and rest it on the clean towel.

☐	Firmly holding onto the drainage tube where it comes out of your chest skin, with your other hand squeeze the tube flat and push your fingers down the tube until you have pushed all the fluid into the drainage bulb at the end. (The tube may stretch slightly while you're doing this.)
☐	If your drain has volumes marked on it, hold it up to your eye level and make a note of how much fluid you measure. If you're using a measuring cup, squeeze the fluid from the drain into the cup without leaving any fluid in the drain. Be sure to mark down the amount measured on your log sheet, as this will determine how quickly the surgeon can remove the drain.
☐	Open your drain and pour the fluid down the toilet.
☐	With the drain still open, fold it over on itself to flatten it, and squeeze it to press out as much air as possible. Put the cap back on, and then let the drain unfold. (Doing this creates suction that helps suck the extra fluid from your surgical wound.)
☐	Pin or place the drain back in place.
☐	If you used a measuring cup, rinse and dry it.
☐	Repeat this procedure till you have emptied all the drains.

☐	Wash your hands again.
☐	If you're finding this hard to visualize, an incredibly helpful woman recorded her drainage tube experiences on YouTube so that you can watch exactly how she does it: *www.youtube.com/watch? v=ORf6AB36Gnc*
☐	Most surgeons will allow you to shower as soon as you're home, but how do you shower with several drainage tubes dangling from your chest? (Keep in mind that you likely won't be able to raise your arms above your head.) The easiest solution is to tie a ribbon (in advance) that can easily go over your head and comes to about chest height, and dangle the drainage tubes through the ribbon while you shower. A spouse's old necktie, or a waterproof waist pouch, can also work.

When to Call Your Doctor

Call your doctor if:

- The drainage tubes fall out
- You run more than 100 degree fever
- The skin is red at the site of the tube
- There's a lot of drainage from the skin around the tube site
- There's tenderness and swelling at the drain site

- The fluid that's draining smells peculiar, is bright red, or looks like pus
- There seems to be a higher volume of fluid draining for more than one day
- There is suddenly no fluid draining
- You experience a severe increase in pain

Fill-in: Drainage Log

Here's a log where you can easily keep track of your drainage measurements. Be sure the drains are labeled A, B, C, D, or 1, 2, 3, 4 so you don't lose track of which is which.

Drainage Log				
Drain #	Date	Time	Amount	Total Over Last 24 Hours
1 (A)				
2 (B)				
3 (C)				
4 (D)				

Drain #	Date	Time	Amount	Total Over Last 24 Hours

Drain #	Date	Time	Amount	Total Over Last 24 Hours

(Bring this log sheet to your follow-up doctor appointment.)

Checklist: Pain Management

✓	Pain Management
☐	Though most women find the pain of mastectomy manageable, people experience different amounts of discomfort after surgery, and recovery will occur faster with good pain control.
☐	You'll have better luck controlling your pain if you take pain medication *before* your discomfort becomes severe.
☐	Unless your doctor tells you otherwise, don't take aspirin (or any non-steroidal anti-inflammatory drug including Advil, Motrin, and Aleve) in the days right after surgery because it interferes with your body's ability to clot blood. Tylenol is ok, however.
☐	Post-surgery pain can persist for much longer than doctors acknowledge—days, weeks, even months are not unusual for some women.
☐	Do not try to manage your pain by consuming alcohol or any drug that's not prescribed by your doctor while you're recovering from surgery; sometimes there are interactions between medications.
☐	Both the surgery and the pain pills can cause constipation. To combat constipation, drink more liquids, eat a high-fiber diet (more prunes and bran and vegetables) and get out of bed and walk around

	as frequently as possible.
☐	If you're experiencing discomfort where you've had lymph nodes removed, try a small pillow under your armpit, or try applying an icepack wrapped in a cloth.
☐	You may have a sore throat for a few days following surgery due to the tube that is customarily inserted down patients' throats during surgery. Ask your doctor if throat lozenges, Xylocaine Viscous (lidocaine viscous), or over the counter pain pills are permissible if your throat is bothering you.
☐	If you've had reconstructive surgery at the same time as a mastectomy, you will likely feel sore (and tired) for at least a week or two; longer if you've had a flap procedure.
☐	One effect of surgery seldom mentioned by doctors is the phenomenon of "phantom itch" that many women experience in the area where nerves were cut in their chest and underarms. Similar to amputees' phantom limb pain, phantom itch can't be effectively scratched. Sometimes scratching *around* the itching area provides relief. Phantom itch can last for years after surgery.

The Post-Surgery Doctor Appointment Checklist

ଔ ଓ

A week or two after your surgery, you'll have the opportunity to sit down with your surgeon or oncologist to hear about his/her findings (and have your drainage tubes removed.) Although most women who have surgery go on to a combination of chemotherapy and/or radiation, treatment protocols differ depending on what the surgeon found.

Careful readers will notice that some of these questions are repeated from the *Make Some Medical Decisions* chapter (p. 33). Although all of these questions are worth asking pre-surgery, surgeons won't always be able to definitively tell you some of this information until after they see the pathology report (such as which stage or grade your cancer is, or whether it has spread to lymph nodes); other times, doctors are reluctant to burden you with too many details up front. So we've repeated the relevant questions here, just to make sure that you don't miss getting the answers you need.

Here's what to ask your surgeon:

Fill-in: What's Next After Surgery?

What's Next After Surgery?	
What type of breast cancer do I have?	
What stage of breast cancer do I have?	
What grade of breast cancer do I have?	
Can you explain my pathology report?	
Has my cancer spread to lymph nodes (how many?) or other organs?	
Do I have estrogen- or progesterone-positive tumors, and what does that mean in terms of treatment?	
Do I have HER2/neu-positive tumors, and what does that mean in terms of treatment?	
If I'm HER2/neu-positive and you're recommending Herceptin, am I a candidate	

for the T-DM1 antibody-drug conjugate? (See p. 240)	
Should I get a 2nd opinion on the tissue samples?	
Do I need other tests before we decide on treatment?	
What are my options for treatment?	
What treatment is most appropriate for me? Why?	
What will treatment involve, and where will it be done? Will I need chemotherapy? Radiation therapy?	
If you're recommending chemotherapy, can I get a referral to have a baseline bone density scan before I begin? (See p. 331)	
What are the short and long-term side-effects of the treatment?	
Can we do anything to prevent	

the side-effects?	
What are my odds of recurrence with the treatment you've outlined?	
What will the day-to-day effects on my life be of this treatment? What changes should I expect to make? What will my energy level be? Can I / should I exercise? Will I be able to work during treatment? Travel?	
Will I go through menopause as a result of treatment?	
Will I be able to have children after treatment?	
Should I get genetic testing?	
Should I look into clinical trials? (See p. 277)	
What can I do to prepare for treatment?	
Should I change my diet?	
What type of follow-up will I	

need long-term?	
Can I schedule my treatment around my work commitments?	
Can I get a prescription (for insurance reimbursement) for a prosthesis and mastectomy bra?	
Is it worth getting an MRI after a lumpectomy? (Some radiation oncologists feel that mammograms don't reveal small areas of residual disease post-surgery.)	

Record results of your surgeries in the appendices *Surgery Record* (p. 321) and *Treatment Summary* (p. 315).

The Infusion Port Checklist

☙ ❧

*T*hey *tell you that nobody will be able to see your infusion port. That's what they tell you. Right. You can't see it. If you're blind. Or if it's dark. Otherwise you can see it just fine—it looks like a small remote control unit buried in the skin under your collar bone.*

Rather than subject your veins to the continued pokes of blood tests and IV insertions involved in chemotherapy, and particularly if you've had lymph nodes removed and are at risk for lymphedema in both arms, your doctor may suggest an infusion port, also called a Port-A-Cath, to avoid vein collapse.

The port is surgically implanted under the skin in your upper chest, usually on the right side; once implanted, it will look like a small (marble-sized) bump under your skin. It provides internal access to a large vein through which they'll give your chemotherapy (and also draw blood, etc.) Since it's internal, it presents no problem to bathe or swim.

The procedure takes no more than 30 minutes, and is done as outpatient surgery, usually with sedation and local anesthesia (though you can ask to skip the sedation); you'll probably be permitted to leave the hospital an hour or two later.

Checklist: Infusion Port Surgery

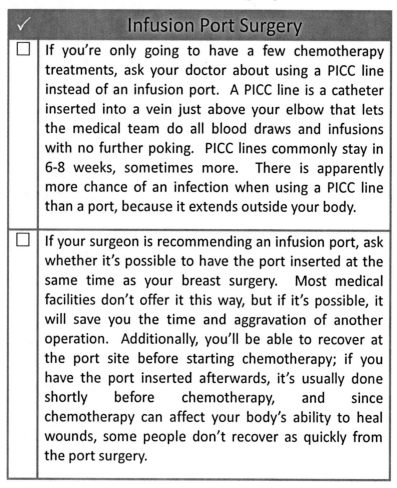

✓	Infusion Port Surgery
☐	If you're only going to have a few chemotherapy treatments, ask your doctor about using a PICC line instead of an infusion port. A PICC line is a catheter inserted into a vein just above your elbow that lets the medical team do all blood draws and infusions with no further poking. PICC lines commonly stay in 6-8 weeks, sometimes more. There is apparently more chance of an infection when using a PICC line than a port, because it extends outside your body.
☐	If your surgeon is recommending an infusion port, ask whether it's possible to have the port inserted at the same time as your breast surgery. Most medical facilities don't offer it this way, but if it's possible, it will save you the time and aggravation of another operation. Additionally, you'll be able to recover at the port site before starting chemotherapy; if you have the port inserted afterwards, it's usually done shortly before chemotherapy, and since chemotherapy can affect your body's ability to heal wounds, some people don't recover as quickly from the port surgery.

☐	Avoid food and beverages the day of the procedure (until after you're done with the surgery).
☐	Avoid aspirin (or any non-steroidal anti-inflammatory drug including Advil, Motrin, and Aleve) in the days before and after surgery because it interferes with your body's ability to clot blood. Tylenol is ok, however.

Using Your Infusion Port

- Before going for each chemotherapy treatment, your doctor will probably recommend that you apply a topical anesthetic (such as EMLA) to the port site, taped over with Tegaderm (a clear bandage) about an hour before your scheduled chemotherapy treatment. When they insert the IV (or draw blood) this will cause the needle insertion into the port to be relatively painless.

- Even after chemotherapy ends, most women keep the infusion port in place for the period during which they get Herceptin.

- If the port will be unused for a period of time, it must be flushed monthly with a saline solution to prevent infection.

- When your IV treatments end, the infusion port can be surgically removed (in a day surgery procedure similar to insertion).

The Prosthesis Checklist

❦ ❧

External prostheses, also called breast forms, are put inside a bra to make your breasts look natural, and are used by women who have decided not to have reconstruction, or who are waiting for their reconstruction. Even women who have had reconstruction may need partial prostheses and mastectomy bras.

Checklist: Prostheses

✓	Prostheses
☐	Before you shop for a prosthesis, ask your doctor to write you a prescription for both a prosthesis and a prosthetic bra, so that you can (possibly) get insurance reimbursement.
☐	Prostheses are sold in surgical supply stores, lingerie shops, and in the lingerie departments of many department stores.
☐	Call before you go to make sure that a professional prosthesis fitter will be there.

☐	Bring your partner or a friend with you when you shop; it can be overwhelming (and demoralizing) to shop for a prosthesis.
☐	Wear a form-fitting top, so that you can see how the various prostheses look when you move.
☐	Try on different types of prostheses: They vary in weight, shape, and consistency. Custom-made prostheses are also available.
☐	Prostheses may feel heavy, but they should also feel comfortable and should stay in place when you move.
☐	Ask if the prosthesis will absorb perspiration, and how you should care for it.
☐	Keep the following points in mind: • Prostheses are designed to fit in special bras made with pockets • Experts recommend fitting the bra first, and only then identifying the size prosthesis that looks best on you. • If you already have a favorite bra, you can also have it fitted with a pocket. • If you don't like the 'slipping up' feeling of a bra, try a camisole with a pocketed shelf bra.

- Silicone breast forms are the most popular type of form, and are the most lifelike. Their key disadvantage is that they're heavy (though now all the manufacturers have introduced lighter-weight forms.) They can also cause perspiration (though many are now being made with moisture-wicking backing.) Attachable silicone breast forms, which take the weight off your shoulder, are also available; these can be worn with a regular (unpocketed) bra. Silicone breast forms run $200 to $400 for a pair.

    o Amoena, American Breast Care, Classique, Jodee, Nearly Me, Silique, and Trulife all make silicone breast forms.

- Non-silicone breast forms are less popular, though they're very lightweight (i.e., more comfortable.) They don't have the lifelike feel of the silicone breast forms.

- Fabric breast forms are also available: For $65 to $85 you can get custom knitted cotton and cashmere forms in a variety of styles from *www.titbits.ca/v1/tb_shop.html*.

- For swimming, there are special non-silicone breast forms; or try an (almost weightless) netted bath "poof" or "loofah" (used for shower exfoliation) which will dry quickly.

www.Anita.com/de-en/Products,Anita_care, Swimwear

- Small prostheses ("equalizers") are available for women who have had part of a breast removed (through lumpectomy or a segmental mastectomy).

- External nipple prostheses are also sold to cover flat or missing nipples.

- You can order a prosthesis online (though it might be easier to determine fit in person):

  o Make Me Heal, (866) 363-4325, *www.Make MeHeal.com*
  o Mastectomy Shop, (877) 413-2272, *www. MastectomyShop.com*
  o Nearly You, (866) 722-6168, *www.NearlyYou.com*
  o Nordstrom, (888) 282-6060, *shop.Nordstrom.com/c/prosthesis-program?origin=srcontent*
  o Women's Health Boutique, (800) 525-2420, *www.WHBLongview.com*

☐ Even women who have had reconstruction may find that they need partial prostheses and mastectomy bras.

- One option is to wear what's called 'partial'

shapers on top of the implants, with a mastectomy bra.

- Another option is the new braGGs reconstruction bra, which is designed specifically for women who have had reconstruction. *BraggsOnline.com*

☐ Check out the website *www.BreastFree.org* for useful information on prostheses.

The Chemotherapy Checklist

CƆ ৪০

Half-way through they switch you from AC chemotherapy to Taxol chemotherapy, which is supposed to be 'easier.' Here's what easier entails: They actually make you lie in a bed, because they give you so many antihistamines (to make sure you don't get a fatal allergic reaction to the Taxol) that they're afraid you're so drugged up you'll fall straight out of your chair. Then they tell you that they need to give you the Taxol through fiberglass tubing (rather than plastic) because the Taxol eats straight through the plastic. Oh boy.

Post-surgery, many women will undergo chemotherapy.

- Chemotherapy, cancer-killing drugs usually given intravenously, can take anywhere from half an hour to several hours to administer. It's usually given on an outpatient basis at a hospital, infusion center, or in a doctor's office.

- The treatment spacing (every week, every other week, etc.) varies; the most common protocol is AC (Adriamycin [a trade name for doxorubicin] / Cytoxan [a trade name for cyclophosphamide]) chemotherapy every other week for four treatments, followed by 12 weeks of weekly Taxol (a trade name for paclitaxel). Or, alternatively, the same AC schedule (every other week for four treatments) but followed by four large doses of Taxol, one every other week. Triple-negative women often receive a variation of this involving fluorouracil, epirubicin, and/or docetaxel (see p. 263 for more information on triple-negative breast-cancer).

- If you're HER2/neu-positive, ask your doctor if you are a candidate for the T-DM1 antibody drug conjugate, or other targeted therapies.

- You can usually arrange the treatment dates in advance so that you'll be able to plan your work and home schedules.

- Before administering chemotherapy each treatment, nurses will draw your blood (either intravenously, or through your port) to make sure your white blood cell count has rebounded to a normal level since the last treatment; if it hasn't, your immune system isn't strong enough for more chemotherapy, and you'll be rescheduled.

- Doctors often recommend Neulastim (or Neulasta or Imupeg—all are trade names for pegfilgrastim) injections the day after each AC treatment to bolster your white blood counts.

The more organized and prepared for chemotherapy you are, the easier your experience is likely to be. Here are some suggestions:

Checklist: Treatment Day

✓	Treatment Day
☐	Eat before you go. You'll experience no (or less) nausea if you eat a **whole-grain** meal about two hours before your treatment.
☐	**Reduce fats and sugars** to lessen the risk of nausea.
☐	**Don't eat your favorite foods** before a treatment— you may end up with unpleasant associations between your food and the treatment.
☐	Remember to **drink** a lot to get those toxins flushing through your system quickly.
☐	Sucking on a **peppermint** candy during treatment may help if your mouth tastes unpleasant.
☐	Wear **comfortable clothing** and comfortable shoes to treatments. If you have a port, wear a (button-down) shirt so that the port can be easily accessed. Bring a sweater or jacket, and warm socks, because hospitals are often chilly.
☐	Bring a **book** or relaxation tape so you have something to do while waiting.
☐	Bring a **snack** (carbohydrates such as bread or crackers are usually best) and water.

☐	**Something cold** to snack on (popsicles, ice chips, etc.) can help prevent mouth sores, one of the possible side-effects of chemotherapy (particularly if you're taking Adriamycin.)
☐	Ask a nurse whether you should plunge your fingers in ice water or wear ice mitts during AC treatment to prevent nail problems.
☐	Don't forget your **calendar** (for scheduling future appointments and timing and dosage details of medications) and medical records.
☐	Bring a **friend.** You'll likely be spending hours in the chemotherapy room, and you can have some nice, uninterrupted time with someone you love, or with someone you'd like to get to know better. Also, you'll need someone to drive you home; your response to treatment will vary, and you might not be physically capable of driving yourself home.
☐	If nausea is a problem, try placing an **acupressure band** on your wrist a few hours before chemotherapy.
☐	Ask for a heated blanket, which some women find makes them feel much happier during treatments, particularly in frosty hospitals.
☐	The chemotherapy drug Adriamycin is a red color; if your urine is red afterwards, it's not a cause for concern.

Checklist: Other Chemotherapy Tips

✓	Other Chemotherapy Tips
☐	Nausea, fatigue, and hair loss are the most common chemotherapy side-effects. The best treatment for fatigue and exhaustion, and a good treatment for nausea as well, is moderate exercise.
☐	Wash your hands often—and make everyone else wash theirs. Use an antibacterial cleaner, and make family members (and guests) use it too. Bring wipes with you when you leave the house, so that you can easily clean your hands wherever you go without having to share a communal towel.
☐	Face mask. If you're going to be in a crowded venue such as a concert hall or church or synagogue, consider wearing a face mask. It may not totally prevent you from getting sick, but it will at least prevent egregious cheek-kissers from getting too close.
☐	Moisturize at least twice daily (with a moisturizer for sensitive skin) to avoid skin dryness. Chemotherapy drugs will dry out your skin, and you don't want to inadvertently scratch and possibly cause an infection. After showering, pat yourself dry (don't rub—that also can lead to infection) and moisturize immediately.
☐	Be sure you're not over-showering—you don't want

212 The Chemotherapy Checklist

	to strip away too much moisture.
☐	If you don't have a port, your fingers or arms will feel particularly sensitive because of the constant poking, so be sure you coat them with Vaseline or moisturizer every day. Use a fragrance-free product, because the chemotherapy will heighten your sense of smell.
☐	Chemotherapy makes you photosensitive, so avoid the sun: A rash or sunburn may cause infection (and can also contribute to lymphedema). Wear double your usual sunscreen SPF, cover up with tightly knit cotton clothing, and limit your sun time.
☐	Schedule preferred time for visitors. Your friends will want to drop by to show support, but if you've just come back from a treatment and are throwing up into the sink, you'd probably rather not see them. Figure out what timing works best for you, and ask friends to visit when you'll enjoy them.
☐	Be sure that you're not over-scheduling visitors; your energy level will likely be depleted, and even incredibly social people (like me!) find that two or three visitors a day is probably more than sufficient. When you've had enough visitors, post a polite note on your front door that advises people to come another time. *Hi! I'm having my post-chemotherapy nap at the moment—mornings are a great time to come by and*

	visit! I'll look forward to seeing you soon!
☐	Nap during the day. You'll likely find it difficult to sleep as well as you used to at night, and you'll be more fatigued because of the treatment, so schedule yourself so that you can nap mid-day—and then be sure you nap during that time, rather than checking email or leafing through the newspaper.
☐	If you're planning to follow a special diet during chemotherapy (see p. 81), have your family help in keeping an up-to-date shopping list. When you run out of ingredients, you can just circle them on your list, and when a friendly visitor offers to help you can send them off with the list. (A sample grocery list is in the appendix on p. 292.)
☐	To make sure your chemotherapy is providing optimal benefits to your body, with minimal undesired side-effects, be sure you visualize the chemotherapy as a friend: Think, "Thank goodness for this chemotherapy, which is making my body strong and powerful; I feel rested and great after the treatment" (rather than, "I hate this chemotherapy, it makes me feel horrible and nauseated.") (See p. 139 for more on guided visualization for chemotherapy.)
☐	On chemotherapy treatment day, and for several days thereafter, drink ten glasses of water each day (but not during, or immediately after, meals.)

☐	Exercise daily, even if it's only a ten-minute walk.
☐	Ask for help in lifting heavy items (particularly food items that may be hot); the chemotherapy can numb your fingers, and some women complain about dropping things.
☐	Before starting or continuing vitamins during chemotherapy, speak to your oncologist. Some doctors advocate taking vitamins for nutritional supplementation; others are concerned that antioxidant vitamins are detrimental during chemotherapy, because they may accelerate the growth of certain cancers.
☐	In particular, avoid grapefruit and echinacea during chemotherapy, both of which can interfere with the body's ability to absorb the chemotherapy drugs.
☐	Some nausea during chemotherapy can be unavoidable, but if you're throwing up, talk to your doctor: drugs can prevent it. Particularly if you're on AC, ask about adding Emend, a steroid, and Zofran to your regimen. (Emend is a particularly expensive drug, so some doctors don't prescribe it initially, but if you're suffering, *ask*.)
☐	If you're suffering from constipation, add more fiber to your diet. If that doesn't work, try Metamucil. If you're still suffering, ask your doctor about docusate sodium (an over-the-counter stool softener.) Some

	women find sesame oil helps with constipation.
☐	If you're suffering from diarrhea, try avoiding lactose (dairy).
☐	You might also want to invest in pair of pants with a soft elastic waist, so that you won't need to struggle with buttons or zippers if you're spending a lot of time rushing to the bathroom.
☐	If you have acid reflux, ask your doctor about taking an antacid. You can also try a teaspoon of baking soda in warm water.
☐	If you've got dry mouth, and especially if you're starting to get mouth sores, ask your doctor about taking Biotene; it's available as mouthwash, toothpaste, and/or chewing gum. Peridex is also effective.
☐	If you get thrush (an oral yeast infection) from the chemotherapy, some women suggest baking soda (try a teaspoon in warm water). Other women find that coconut oil relieves thrush. (You can purchase coconut oil at most health food stores.)
☐	Some women find that the steroids administered during chemotherapy will make sleep difficult, and suggest (controlled-release) Ambien. Check with your doctor first.

☐	If you're getting Neulastim (Neulasta, Imupeg, pegfilgrastim) to boost your white blood count, you can get bone pain as a result. Joint pain, muscle pain, nausea, and headache are other common side-effects associated with Neulastim. Ask your doctor if there's any problem with taking painkiller half an hour before each injection (and for one to two days afterwards.) Most women find that Aleve or Motrin work best; some women also find Claritin (an allergy medicine) to be effective.
☐	Remember to purchase (and use) new cosmetics: outdated cosmetics can cause infection.
☐	If you want to get a manicure or pedicure, bring your own equipment to prevent infection. Nail polish enhanced with silicium is helpful for overall nail health, if you're going to use nail polish. If your fingernails are discoloring, try wearing ice mitts during treatment. Tea tree oil (applied topically) can also help.
☐	Get a warm cap in which you can sleep comfortably. If you can find a cap that is seam-free, it will be more comfortable.
☐	If you had radiation *prior to* chemotherapy, be alert for 'radiation recall,' where the irradiated area turns red and irritated as it was during radiation; this can be caused by chemotherapy drugs. Tell your doctor.

☐ Echocardiogram: If your doctor is planning on AC as part of your chemotherapy regimen, and particularly if you'll be getting Herceptin, too, you'll probably be sent for an echocardiogram (heart ultrasound) every two or three months, to check for heart damage. The procedure takes no more than 20 minutes, and is done in a doctor's office or hospital. It involves only the removal of your shirt so that they can rub the ultrasound probe over your chest. It's entirely painless.

☐ Notify your doctor if you've never had chicken pox, and come into contact with either chicken pox or shingles.

☐ Do not become pregnant during chemotherapy. Despite menopausal symptoms, it's possible (and dangerous to the baby) to become pregnant.

Checklist: Managing Nausea

Chemotherapy-induced nausea is one of the biggest problems—and biggest fears—of those facing cancer treatment. Here are some ways to alleviate nausea:

✓	Managing Nausea
☐	Instead of three large meals per day, try five or six smaller meals.
☐	Avoid beverages with meals, or in the two hours after eating, to prevent nausea. (But drink the rest of the day so you don't get dehydrated.) When you drink, drink slowly.
☐	First thing in the morning, and at the first hint of nausea, eat dry foods—toast or crackers.
☐	Low fat foods are better than greasy, sugary, or fatty foods; dry foods (toast, crackers) are best. Salty foods will likely go down better than sweet foods. Chew food thoroughly.
☐	For two hours immediately after eating, do not lie down. (Sleeping sitting up is fine.)
☐	Fresh air or loose clothing can help control nausea. Or try accupressure (seasick) wrist-bands. Hypnosis has also proven helpful to some.

☐	Have someone else prepare your meals, or prepare your meals ahead of time.
☐	Avoid cooking odors, and being around cooking preparation. Perfume and smoke odor can also contribute to nausea.
☐	Consuming cold liquids, salty liquids, ice chips, or ginger, and an icepack on the back of your neck, can all help relieve nausea.
☐	Use plastic eating utensils, rather than metal silverware, which (oddly) can set off nausea.
☐	Ginger and ginger tea have been shown to be effective in combating nausea, but be careful not to take ginger when chemotherapy lowers your platelet count, because of its anticoagulant effect. Check with your doctor to be sure.
☐	Some women find lemon (either fresh lemon, squeezed into water, lemon drops, or lemon oil to sniff) helpful for queasiness.
☐	Relaxation exercises can help.

Checklist: Hair Loss

During chemotherapy you're likely to lose most of your scalp hair, and possibly all of your body and facial hair as well. Here are some things to consider:

✓	Hair Loss
☐	Hair loss that you experience during chemotherapy is temporary; after you stop the chemotherapy, your hair will start to regrow (though the texture and color may be slightly different than the hair you lost.)
☐	Hair loss usually begins within two to three weeks of starting chemotherapy.
☐	For facial hair, get an eyeliner pencil so that you can draw in your eyebrows when that hair falls out.
☐	Have someone snap a close-up photo of your face that you can use as a reference in drawing on eyebrows post hair loss.
☐	The glue in fake eyelashes can cause infections, so just use a dark eyeliner pencil around your eyes and skip the falsies.
☐	When your hair starts to fall out in clumps, it might be easier to have your partner or a friend shave the rest of it off entirely; it's demoralizing to see it falling all out over your pillow.

- ☐ Even though you're losing your hair, you should still shampoo your scalp at least once a week to keep it fresh. (Use a baby shampoo—because of chemotherapy you'll have no natural hair oils, so you need a gentle shampoo.)

- ☐ Silk scarves are likely to slip off your head without hair to keep them in place; cotton is a better choice.

- ☐ If you're going for a wig, buying it when you still have your hair will help them match the color and style more easily.

- ☐ A human hair wig will be lighter and more comfortable than a synthetic wig (but more expensive). A synthetic wig won't last as long as a human hair wig (but even a synthetic wig will last at least a year).

- ☐ Shampoo, condition, and air-dry your wig. Or you can use a blow-dryer until the wig is almost dry; then air-dry the rest of the way.

- ☐ Plastic-bristled brushes work best on wigs.

- ☐ Keep the wig on a wig stand when you're not wearing it to keep the shape. You might want to cover it with a scarf to keep it dust-free.

	A wig-liner worn under the wig will help keep the wig from getting itchy. (If you can't find a wig-liner, cut the middle part from a pair of pantyhose and use that.)
	For details of where to purchase wigs and scarves, see p. 108.

Chemotherapy Side-Effects

While chemotherapy kill cancer cells, it also damages some normal cells, which leads to all sorts of side-effects. Record any side-effects you experience in your log (see p. 226), so that your doctor will know how to adjust your medication if necessary. Many side-effects will disappear entirely once you're done with treatment. Common side-effects include:

- Nausea
- Exhaustion
- Mouth sores
- Appetite changes
- Diarrhea
- Skin pigmentation changes
- Hair loss
- Low blood counts
- Easy bruising or bleeding
- Metallic mouth taste
- High risk of infection

- Irregularities in menstrual cycle (along with possible early onset of menopause)

- Nails: Both fingernails and toenails may become weak, brittle, deformed, turn dark and even fall off. Avoid manicures, pedicures, or cutting your cuticles, which could increase the risk of infection. You should also avoid using artificial nails. Nails usually grow back within about 6 months after treatment.

- Dry eyes: Chemotherapy can make your corneas red and dry. Ask your doctor about eye drops.

- Some women experience faintness, dizziness, and sweating.

- 'Chemo brain,' a slight or major change in concentration, memory, and attention. It often lasts well after chemotherapy has ended, though it eventually goes away for most women.

When to Call Your Doctor

Particular side-effects to watch for and notify your doctor about:

- Rashes: During chemotherapy, if a skin rash appears, call your doctor immediately. Rashes can signal a reaction to your drugs, or an infection that needs to be treated.

- Bruising: If you spot bruises (without having bumped into something), call your doctor immediately. Your platelet count may be too low, possibly requiring a blood transfusion. (Minor spotty changes in pigmentation, on the other hand, are likely to be responses to the chemotherapy chemicals, and will fade once treatment is complete.)

- Fever: Your doctor will tell you how high the thermometer can go before you call him, so be sure to take your temperature if you're at all warm. Fevers may require hospitalization.

- Some women experience what's called 'hand-foot syndrome' with redness, swelling, and blistering on the palms and soles. Inform your doctor.

- One side-effect to be particularly alert for is neuropathy, or nerve damage (also called CIPN, chemotherapy-induced peripheral neuropathy). Many women experience the onset of neuropathy (numbness, tingling, burning, faintness, dizziness, sweating, or pain in the hands and feet) particularly during Taxol treatments. If you suspect neuropathy, *tell your oncologist immediately*: Neuropathy can worsen with continued treatments, and partial paralysis is a fear.

  o Some women suffering from neuropathy are helped by vitamin E, calcium, magnesium, and Neurontin (which, however, includes memory loss as a possible side-effect). Women report that alcohol and sugar seem to worsen neuropathy. Ask your doctor.

o A study in the Journal of the Society for Integrative Oncology suggests acupuncture as a possible remedy for chemotherapy-induced neuropathy.

o Consider contacting The Neuropathy Association, (212) 692-0662, *www.Neuropathy.org*.

- If you're getting Neulastim (Neulasta, Imupeg, pegfilgrastim) injections and you experience any of the following, head to the emergency room:

o Sudden signs of allergy (rash, hives, swelling, difficulty breathing)

o Pain in your upper left abdomen

- Rarely, women experience blood clots as a side-effect of chemotherapy, usually in the legs. Contact your doctor immediately if you experience unexplained swelling or discomfort in your calf muscles.

Fill-in: Chemotherapy Log

Chemotherapy Log	
Date	Side-Effect

Date	Side-Effect

Record details of your overall chemotherapy regimen in the appendix *Treatment Summary*, p. 315, and details of your doctor visits in *Doctor Appointments*, p. 333. Details of your chemotherapy side-effects can be recorded in the *Chemotherapy Log* above.

The Radiation Checklist

It seems just a little ironic to be having endless conversations about the desirability of getting a lead case for my cell phone so that it won't be emitting radiation, while at the same time undergoing radiation of a much higher strength. On purpose.

If you've had a lumpectomy, or you've had a mastectomy with lymph nodes affected, or your tumor is particularly large and they would like to shrink it before surgery, you'll probably need radiation, that is, treatment with high-energy x-rays. Radiation therapy can reduce recurrence rates by as much as 50%. Usually when your doctor says you'll need radiation, he's referring to *external beam radiation*. In some cases, your doctor will prescribe internal radiation therapy called *brachytherapy*, which also goes by brand names such as MammoSite.

Compared to chemotherapy, radiation therapy for most women is a piece of cake. Radiation treatment itself is painless.

External Beam Radiation Overview

- Treatment is usually in an outpatient center, and takes just a few minutes each day. During each treatment you are exposed to a beam of high-energy x-rays generated by a machine called a linear accelerator.

- Unlike chemotherapy, treatment is usually given five days a week, for three to eight weeks; most women have five week protocols.

- If your oncologist is recommending Tamoxifen (see p. 243), ask about starting Tamoxifen during radiation treatments: some radiation oncologists think combining Tamoxifen with radiation treatment is most effective; others think that Tamoxifen can desensitize the cells to radiation therapy, thus making it less effective.

- Common side-effects, which are cumulative, are sunburn, exhaustion, and an increased risk of lymphedema (long-term arm swelling).

- At your first appointment, the doctors will do what's referred to as a 'simulation' where they pinpoint exactly where on your chest they'll need to direct the high-energy radiation.

- The simulation will take approximately 45 minutes. They'll immobilize you in some sort of brace or restrictive equipment (the exact immobilization device differs from hospital to hospital) so that you can't move. Then they'll take a series of x-rays from different angles.

- In most of the U.S., the procedure involves applying a small tattoo to your chest so that the technicians can later zero in on the exact spot to be irradiated; in some parts of the U.S. and many other countries they use colored magic markers. The advantage of the tattoo is that it's discreet; the advantages of the markers are that they are not permanent (you can wash them off when you are done with radiation), there's no pain involved in applying them, and there's no problem with future MRIs.

- Lead shields: There is some speculation in the cancer discussion forums online about whether women should be wearing lead shields during radiation procedures, to protect body parts that don't need irradiation (much like the reason for the lead aprons you don in the dentist's office.) In fact, the external beam radiation used for breast cancer treatments is of such high energy that it totally penetrates the lead apron anyway, so there's no advantage in doing this. This may not be true for other types of cancer and radiation, but for breast cancer external beam radiation, oncologists don't advise using lead shields. Your oncologist may shield you during brachytherapy, however.

Internal Radiation Therapy Overview

- For early-stage lumpectomies, your doctor might prescribe *brachytherapy*, also called *balloon catheter radiation*. You might be eligible for brachytherapy if:

  o You're scheduled for a lumpectomy

  o You have no lymph node involvement

  o You're at least 45 years old; some oncologists say you have to be at least 60 years old

  o Your tumor is no more than 3 cm in diameter

  o You can leave at least 7 millimeters of tissue between your skin and the balloon catheter

- In brachytherapy, a balloon catheter is placed in the lumpectomy cavity, and filled with saline (salt-water) solution from the other end, which remains outside the breast; the catheter is either inserted during the lumpectomy, or later in a separate procedure.

- Treatment is usually given twice a day for five days.

- In each treatment, a small radioactive pellet or "seed" is inserted through the catheter by a computer-controlled machine for a few minutes, delivering a carefully-measured dose of radiation directly to the tumor area. (In some brachytherapy systems, a tiny high-energy x-ray source is used instead of the radioactive pellet.)

- After the five-day treatment, the balloon is drained and then removed.

- Your breast will avoid the "sunburning" of external beam radiation.

- Healthy breast tissue will not be irradiated.

- It involves less fatigue than external beam radiation.

- Some women complain that the saline balloon feels peculiar.

- Infections around the catheter site are possible; you may experience redness, bruising, pain, and drainage.

- There is little local recurrence reported after brachytherapy.

- The procedure is usually covered by insurance.

- In a recent study, brachytherapy was associated with a 17% higher rate of wound and skin complications in the year after treatment, compared to whole breast irradiation.

Checklist: Radiation

✓	Radiation
☐	If you're getting a tattoo: Be sure to ask your doctor if the tattoo contains metal. Older tattoo technology, which is still occasionally used for radiation marking in the U.S., involves metal. Once you've had a metal tattoo inserted, you may need to take extra precautions when getting an MRI in the future.
☐	If you received the magic markers instead of the tattoo, keep in mind that while water is fine, you should avoid ferocious scrubbing as well as the use of soap on your chest, so as not to obliterate your radiation guidelines. If the lines seem to be fading, be sure to tell your technician at your next appointment, so that the lines can be re-drawn.
☐	Use only baby soap to wash the radiation areas, and avoid scrubbing; your skin will be highly prone to irritation, and the less you do to further irritate it, the better.
☐	Despite the preponderance of online forums recommending various cosmetics for sunburn discomfort experienced by many women during radiation, most doctors actually recommend avoiding soap, alcohol-based products, and all lotions on your chest area during the several weeks of radiation, as

	these can affect the radiation dose you receive.
☐	Be sure to cover up your chest area thoroughly before going outside, even on a cloudy or rainy day, to prevent sun on your radiation areas. That means you need to be extra-careful outside, and particularly at places like the beach.
☐	Ask your doctor about swimming during radiation. Most medical establishments advise that radiation patients **not** engage in swimming during the course of their radiation because swimming in chlorinated water will further dry out the skin.
☐	Be sure you're showering (without soap) twice a day, for at least five minutes, in warm water during each day you're getting radiation treatments. This will go a long way towards helping to avoid skin irritations and burns associated with radiation therapy.
☐	Don't ingest antioxidant supplements during radiation. Antioxidants protect cells from harm—and the whole point of radiation is to damage the cancer cells permanently. By taking antioxidants during radiation, you might inadvertently negate the effect of the radiation. So wait until after treatment to load up on antioxidants.
☐	As with chemotherapy, be sure that during the radiation you're feeding back messages of happiness and strength: "The radiation is making my body strong

and powerful, and I'm going to be healthy as a result" (rather than, "The radiation is making me miserable and it hurts.") The mind/body effect of the positive messaging can be dramatic.

Checklist: Post-Radiation

✓	Post-Radiation
☐	If your skin becomes irritated or burnt during the radiation, doctors recommend that you not swim for at least one month after the irritation fades.
☐	Don't sunbathe for two to three months after the end of your radiation. Avoid exposing your radiated areas to the sun even for short periods of time for several months after radiation ends.
☐	Be alert for 'radiation recall', in which some radiation side-effects (redness, skin irritation, etc.) reappear. Radiation recall can be triggered by both chemotherapy and Tamoxifen.

Fill-in: Radiation Log

Record any side-effects you experience during radiation treatments here:

Date	Side-Effect
Radiation Log	

Date	Side-Effect

Record details of your radiation regimen in the *Radiation Log* above, in the appendix *Treatment Summary* (p. 315), and details of radiation oncology and radiology doctor visits in *Doctor Appointments* (p. 333).

The Herceptin Checklist

ೞ ೞ

Most women who are diagnosed with HER2/neu-positive cancer will be advised to receive *Herceptin* (a trade name for trastuzumab) during, and usually for a year following, chemotherapy treatments.

Herceptin Overview

- Herceptin is a biological therapy; it is not chemotherapy.

- Like chemotherapy, Herceptin is given via IV.

- It is usually given once every three weeks (though it can also be administered every week).

- Side-effects include nausea, vomiting, diarrhea, headache, dry eyes, joint pain, skin rash, cough, fever, chills, weakness, and shortness of breath.

- A more serious possible side-effect is heart disease.

- There are other drugs now being studied that may have beneficial effects similar to Herceptin, so ask your doctor what the latest research indicates and whether

Herceptin is your best option. In clinical trials now is a new drug, T-DM1, which attaches Herceptin to a chemotherapy drug to deliver the chemotherapy only to HER2/neu-positive cancer cells, eliminating many of the side-effects of traditional chemotherapy. Check with your doctor to see if you're a candidate for this.

If you're receiving Herceptin you should also consider adding the following items to your diet as much as possible, all of which have been found to inhibit the growth of HER2/neu-positive cancer. Eat:

- peppers
- cabbage
- celery
- flaxseed oil
- ginger
- green tea
- mackerel
- olive oil
- parsley
- pomegranates
- salmon
- sardines
- turmeric
- walnuts

Echocardiogram: If your doctor is planning on Herceptin as part of your treatment, you'll probably be sent for an echocardiogram (heart ultrasound) every two or three months, as a side-effect of this drug can include problems with a heart valve. The procedure takes no more than 20 minutes, and is done in a doctor's office or hospital. It involves only the removal of your shirt so that they can rub the ultrasound probe over your chest. It's entirely painless.

Fill-in: Herceptin Log

Herceptin Log	
Date	**Side-Effect**

Date	Side-Effect

The Tamoxifen Checklist

CR RD

Breast cancer patients who are *pre*-menopausal and who test positive for estrogen-receptive tumors, or patients (either pre- or post-menopausal) with DCIS (Ductal Carcinoma In Situ, a non-invasive cancer that starts in the milk ducts) are often prescribed Tamoxifen (sold under various trade names including Nolvadex, Istubal, and Valodex; there is also a related drug, Toremifene). Tamoxifen is a pill to block estrogen, and is taken orally, daily, for up to five years (or until menopause).

Tamoxifen Overview

- Tamoxifen reportedly reduces local recurrence, distant recurrence, and new breast cancer rates, for an estimated 10-15 years.

- You can take Tamoxifen with or without food/drink.

- If you'll be having radiation, ask your radiation oncologist about starting Tamoxifen during radiation treatments: some radiation oncologists think combining Tamoxifen with radiation treatment is most effective; others think that Tamoxifen can desensitize the cells to radiation therapy, thus making it less effective.

- According to the American Cancer Society, the genistein in soy can stop Tamoxifen's ability to halt breast cancer growth, so women with estrogen-dependent tumors may want to avoid soy.

- Be alert for 'radiation recall' which can be caused by Tamoxifen; if the area where you had radiation turns irritated and red, notify your doctor.

- If you're taking Tamoxifen, doctors recommend that you avoid the following medicines:

    o Prozac
    o Paxil
    o Cardioquin
    o Wellbutrin
    o Cymbalta
    o Benadryl
    o Mellaril
    o Cordarone
    o Tagamet
    o Zoloft

This is just a short list: there are over 300 drugs that interact with Tamoxifen, so if your doctor prescribes Tamoxifen, be sure to discuss any medications you're already taking, and after you start taking Tamoxifen, be sure to mention it if you are prescribed any additional medications.

- Certain anti-depressants interfere with Tamoxifen. If you're taking anti-depressants, the following information might be important to you.

  Tamoxifen metabolizes (i.e. breaks down in the body) into several important cancer-fighting chemicals, one of which is called CYP2D6; certain anti-depressants interfere with this process. You can have a CYP2D6 blood test, which reveals how well you are metabolizing the Tamoxifen. (This test is not done routinely; insurance may cover it; it costs about $600 otherwise.) For more information, see *medicine.iupui. edu/clinpharm/COBRA/Tamoxifen%20and%202D6v7 .pdf*.

  Effexor, Celexa, and Lexapro are *not* CYP2D6 inhibitors, and are apparently fine while on Tamoxifen, but check with your doctors.

Checklist: Tamoxifen Side-Effects

Tamoxifen comes with its share of side-effects, including night sweats, dry mouth, bloating, nausea, hair thinning, ringing in the ears, fingers freezing in a curled position, achiness, itching, joint pain, fogginess, fatigue, weight gain, hot flashes, mood swings, leg cramps, blood clots, vaginal discharge, vaginal dryness, vaginal bleeding, depression, headaches, cataracts, loss of sex drive, and uterine cancer. Here's how to counter the worst of the symptoms:

✓	Tamoxifen Side-Effects

☐	**For nausea try the following:**
	
	• Take just half of your Tamoxifen pill daily for the first week. After the first week, begin taking the entire pill daily.
	
	    (or)
	
	    Take half of your pill in the morning, and the other half at night, for the first week or two. After that, take your entire pill at the same time each day.
	
	• Take the pill each night just at bedtime. (This will lessen the nausea because you'll have less waking time in which to notice it.)
	
	• You can take the pill with or without food/drink, but take it at the same time each day for maximum efficacy.

☐	**For joint pain** some women report ingesting turmeric helpful.
☐	**For leg cramps**, try: • Altering the time of Tamoxifen ingestion • Daily leg exercises • Aquatic therapy • Drinking sufficient water during the day • Making sure there's enough salt in your diet

	<ul><li>Increasing your potassium intake, e.g. eat more bananas</li><li>Quinine or tonic water or bitter lemon</li><li>Eating just before bed, and/or in the middle of the night</li><li>Keeping your legs warm (i.e. wearing leg-warmers or fuzzy socks)</li></ul>
☐	If you're experiencing **mental fogginess** and **fatigue**, try taking the pill just before bedtime.
☐	If you experience debilitating **hot flashes**, ask your doctor if you're a candidate for Effexor, which is technically an anti-depressant, but is also effective against these Tamoxifen-induced symptoms. You can also try these suggestions: <ul><li>Use layers of clothing and blankets so you can adjust as your temperature changes</li><li>Avoid warm, stuffy rooms</li><li>Avoid spicy foods, large meals, and excess sugar</li><li>Carry a frozen water bottle to keep you cool</li><li>Look into the "Cool Pad" ($119 from *ShieldLife.com*), a mattress pad that cools you down at night</li></ul>
☐	The following suggestions may help you avoid **blood clots**: <ul><li>Some doctors advise, as much as possible,</li></ul>

avoiding crossing your legs while on Tamoxifen.

- Plane flights can be particularly conducive to blood clots. Here are some tricks for plane travel:

  o Wear lymphedema sleeves on your calves during flights. (See the checklist on p. 268 for where to buy lymphedema sleeves for your calves.)
  o Get up and walk around a lot while flying.
  o Take your shoes and socks off.
  o Drink a lot of liquids on the plane.
  o Ask your doctor whether, for a week before the flight and while on the flight, you should take low-dose (81 mg/day) aspirin.

☐ An extremely rare side-effect of Tamoxifen is **uterine cancer**. To be on the safe side, consider the following:

- Whether or not you're post-menopausal, watch for non-menstrual bleeding. If you experience non-menstrual bleeding, head immediately to the emergency room.

- See a gynecologist for a transvaginal/pelvic ultrasound annually to measure the thickness of your endometrium. (Your endometrium will thicken over time, but your gynecologist will be able to determine if it's thickening normally, or should be checked.)

☐ If you don't experience **any** Tamoxifen side-effects, ask your doctor about getting a CYP2D6 test to see if your liver is metabolizing the drug properly; this test is not done routinely, and is usually not covered by insurance.

When to Call Your Doctor

One of Tamoxifen's rare (but still possible) side-effects is thromboembolism, or **blood clots** in the legs.

If you experience the following symptoms, see a doctor immediately:

o   Swelling in the calves

o   Redness in the calves

o   Legs warm to the touch

o   Pain in the calves, like a cramp that won't go away

o   Whether or not you're post-menopausal, watch for non-menstrual bleeding, as it could be a sign of (rare) uterine cancer. If you experience non-menstrual bleeding, head immediately to the emergency room.

Fill-in: Tamoxifen Log

Here you can record your Tamoxifen prescription and any side-effects you experience when taking Tamoxifen:

Tamoxifen Log	
Date	**Drug Name, Dose**
Date	**Side-Effect**

Date	Side-Effect

Date	Side-Effect

The Lupron Checklist

CB EO

B reast cancer patients who are *pre*-menopausal, young, and who test positive for estrogen-receptor-positive tumors are often prescribed Lupron (a trade name for leuprolide acetate), in addition to Tamoxifen, to further slow down the ovaries' estrogen production.

Lupron Overview

- Lupron (and its less prescribed sidekick Zoladex) is usually given by injection once each month (or sometimes every few months), usually for fewer than six months.

- Getting the injection in the buttocks is said to hurt less than receiving it in the arm.

- Lupron can **not** be considered effective birth control.

Checklist: Lupron Side-Effects

✓	Lupron Side-Effects
☐	Side-effects of Lupron include: hot flashes, mood swings, loss of sex drive, osteoporosis, mental fogginess, aggravation of chemotherapy-induced neuropathy, swelling, and weight gain
☐	If you experience debilitating **hot flashes**, try these suggestions: • Use layers of clothing and blankets so you can adjust as your temperature changes • Avoid warm, stuffy rooms • Avoid spicy foods, large meals, and excess sugar • Carry a frozen water bottle to keep you cool • Look into the "Cool Pad" ($119 from *ShieldLife.com*), a mattress pad that cools you down at night
☐	To reduce the risk of **osteoporosis**, some doctors recommend bone-strengthening *bisphosphonates*. Bisphosphonates can cause osteonecrosis of the jaw. To prevent this, some doctors recommend taking *statins* with the bisphosphonates. If your doctor prescribes bisphosphonates for bone health, ask if that's still recommended; the FDA just concluded that bisphosphonates may do more harm than good to women with bone density issues.

Fill-in: Lupron Log

Here you can record your prescription and any side-effects you experience when taking Lupron:

Lupron Log	
Date	**Drug Name, Dose**
Date	**Side-Effect**

Date	Side-Effect

The Aromatase Inhibitors Checklist

℃ℬ ℬↃ

Women who are *post*-menopausal and who test positive for estrogen-receptive tumors are often prescribed *aromatase inhibitors,* which are taken orally daily, for up to five years post-treatment. (Women with DCIS are currently offered only Tamoxifen, whether pre- or post-menopausal.) Aromatase inhibitors stop hormones from turning into estrogen, thus lowering estrogen levels enough that estrogen-sensitive tumors can't grow.

Aromatase Inhibitors Overview

- There are three kinds of aromatase inhibitors prescribed to treat breast cancer:

  o Arimidex (anastrozole)

  o Aromasin (exemestane)

  o Femara (letrozole)

- Aromatase inhibitors are less likely to cause blood clots and uterine cancer than Tamoxifen (which is prescribed primarily for pre-menopausal women).

- Switching to an aromatase inhibitor for 2-3 years (after 2-3 years of Tamoxifen first) seems to convey more benefits than 5 years of Tamoxifen.

- You're likely to experience fewer side-effects if you take the pill with food.

Checklist: Aromatase Inhibitors Side-Effects

Aromatase inhibitors come with their share of side-effects, including hot flashes, vaginal dryness, joint pain, broken bones, osteoporosis, arthritis, night sweats, diarrhea, nausea, bloating, vision problems, fatigue, depression, weight gain, high blood pressure, frequent urination, breast pain or swelling, hair thinning, insomnia, tingling and numbness (similar to carpal tunnel syndrome) in hands and arms, infertility, kidney and liver problems, headaches, mental fogginess, aggravation of chemotherapy-induced neuropathy, and risk of heart problems.

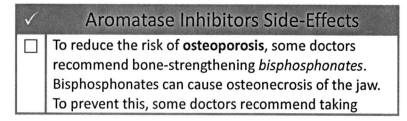

✓	Aromatase Inhibitors Side-Effects
☐	To reduce the risk of **osteoporosis**, some doctors recommend bone-strengthening *bisphosphonates*. Bisphosphonates can cause osteonecrosis of the jaw. To prevent this, some doctors recommend taking

	statins with the bisphosphonates. If your doctor prescribes bisphosphonates for bone health, ask if that's still recommended; the FDA just concluded that bisphosphonates may do more harm than good to women with bone density issues.
☐	If you experience debilitating **hot flashes**, try these suggestions: • Use layers of clothing and blankets so you can adjust as your temperature changes • Avoid warm, stuffy rooms • Avoid spicy foods, large meals, and excess sugar • Carry a frozen water bottle to keep you cool • Look into the "Cool Pad" ($119 from *ShieldLife.com*), a mattress pad that cools you down at night
☐	To forestall **joint pain** and **arthritis**, try eliminating nightshades (potatoes, tomatoes, eggplants, peppers) from your diet. Some women have also reported benefits from (roll-on) topical Capzasin (capsaicin); ask your doctor.
☐	To lessen the problems of **fatigue** and **mental fogginess**, try taking the pills late in the day, before bedtime.

☐	If you are experiencing miserable side-effects, ask your oncologist about switching to a different aromatase inhibitor, which can make a difference.

Fill-in: Aromatase Inhibitors Log

Here you can record any side-effects you experience when taking aromatase inhibitors:

Aromatase Inhibitors Log	
Date	**Drug Name, Dose**
Date	**Side-Effect**

Date	Side-Effect

Date	Side-Effect

The Triple-Negative Checklist

❧ ❧

B etween ten and twenty percent of women diagnosed with breast cancer have what is known as *triple-negative* breast cancer. Triple-negative means that the tumor is estrogen-receptor-negative, progesterone-receptor-negative, and HER2/neu-negative. Women are more likely to be triple-negative if they are:

- Younger than 50

- African American or Latina

- Carrying the BRCA1 (not BRCA2) gene mutations

Women with triple-negative breast cancer face particular challenges.

Triple-negative breast cancer is particularly responsive to chemotherapy (more than other breast cancers), but can not be treated with the rest of the anti-breast cancer arsenal (such as Tamoxifen or aromatase inhibitors, which target estrogen-receptor-positive tumors; or Herceptin, which targets HER2/neu-positive tumors.)

Checklist: Triple-Negative Cancer

✓	Triple-Negative Cancer
☐	Triple-negative cancer tends to be aggressive, but prognosis depends more on the size of the tumor and whether cancer has spread to the lymph nodes than the fact that it is triple-negative per se.
☐	Triple-negative is almost always treated with chemotherapy. The standard protocols include: • AC (Adriamcyin/Cytoxan, that is, doxorubicin with cyclophosphamide) • FAC or CAF, which is AC along with fluorouracil (5FU) • FEC, CEF, or EC, which is a similar protocol with epirubicin (e.g. Ellence) substituted for the doxorubicin • AC-T, AC-D, or TAC, when paclitaxel (Taxol) or docetaxel (Taxotere) is added to AC • FEC-T, when docetaxel (Taxotere) is added to FEC
☐	Studies suggest that a low-fat diet may lower the risk for recurrence after a diagnosis of triple-negative.
☐	Studies show that low vitamin D levels correlate with a higher risk of recurrence for triple-negative women.
☐	Studies suggest that triple-negative is more common in women who use oral contraceptives.

- [ ] The common diabetes drug metformin shows promise in treating triple-negative breast cancer.

- [ ] Triple-negative women who remain disease-free for four years have an extremely low rate of cancer recurrence; after 8 years, the risk falls to almost zero.

- [ ] Post-treatment, triple-negative women see their oncologist every three to six months (for two years), then every six to 12 months (for three or four years), and then once a year. Triple-negative women who had a lumpectomy should get a mammogram or MRI on the remaining breast and breast tissue.

- [ ] A September 2012 comprehensive genetic analysis of breast cancer suggests that there is a stronger connection between triple-negative breast cancer and ovarian cancer than had been previously thought, and therefore that routine treatments for ovarian cancer, such as platinum drugs, as well as new drugs such as PARP inhibitors, might be effective against triple-negative breast cancer.

- [ ] Similarly, because Adriamycin and epirubicin chemotherapy (both of which can cause side-effects such as heart damage) are ineffective against ovarian cancer, researchers are now considering dropping them from the triple-negative treatment protocol.

☐ For more information or support, call the Triple-Negative Helpline at (877) 880-8622.

The Lymphedema Checklist

❦ ❧

Lymphedema is arm swelling caused by improper drainage of lymph fluid. If you've had surgery involving the removal of more than a few lymph nodes from under your arms, and especially if you've also followed up with radiation, you're at high risk for lymphedema. Approximately 30% of women who have axillary lymph node dissection, and even some who don't, will experience lymphedema; the numbers go up in women who've also had radiation.

Lymphedema Overview

- Lymphedema can start soon after surgery and radiation, or it can begin months, sometimes years, later.

- If you're having a full axillary lymph node dissection, ask your doctor for a referral to a physical or occupational therapist for baseline arm measurements pre-surgery. This will enable you to determine later if, and how much, your arms have swollen, so that you can obtain the proper treatment (fill in your baseline measurements in the table on p. 275.)

- If you're ever in a hospital again for surgery, women recommend writing with red magic marker directly on your (affected) arm the words: "Use other arm—no BP, no IV, no sticks on this side" to ensure that medical staff doesn't inadvertently poke the affected arm.

Checklist: Combating Lymphedema

The easiest way to deal with lymphedema is to prevent it from getting out of hand in the first place. Here are things to avoid to help you prevent lymphedema; some of them are easier to avoid than others:

✓	Combating Lymphedema
☐	Moisturize your affected arm(s) daily.
☐	Avoid sunburn. Use SPF-15 or higher sunscreen.
☐	Avoid mosquito and insect bites (wear long sleeves and repellent, etc.) If you are bit or stung, wash the affected area immediately.
☐	Avoid infection.
☐	Keep the affected arm elevated above the heart as much as possible.
☐	Have your blood drawn and shots, vaccines, and IV administered in your unaffected arm (if you have one.)

☐	Have your blood pressure taken on your unaffected arm (if you have one) or on your thigh or leg. (Warn nursing staff that blood pressure taken on legs may measure significantly higher.)
☐	Keep your arm clean.
☐	Wear protective gloves when using chemical cleaners or steel wool, and when doing gardening, yard work, or dishes.
☐	Wear a thimble when sewing to avoid pin pricks.
☐	Use an electric shaver to remove underarm hair; it's less likely to poke you than a safety razor. And use an electric razor, rather than a depilatory.
☐	If you are stung, clean the arm, raise it, and put ice on it. Call your doctor if it becomes infected.
☐	Avoid extreme cold. (Swelling and chapping when you warm up can lead to infection.)
☐	Avoid burns and high heat: Use oven mitts and avoid oil splashes and boiling liquid spills.
☐	Avoid hot tubs, saunas, and heating pads.
☐	Avoid arm constriction: Avoid constricting jewelry, rings, watchbands, clothing, and gloves.

☐	Avoid shoulder straps on briefcases and purses.
☐	Avoid constricting bras. Avoid heavy prostheses.
☐	Avoid heavy lifting with the affected arm. Don't carry heavy packages, suitcases, or even handbags. (See p. 112 for a work-around to a purse.)
☐	Use deodorant rather than antiperspirant (to help keep pores open.)
☐	Avoid cat scratches. (Lymphedema increases your risk of infection in the damaged tissue/extremity.) Apply Betadine or a similar topical antiseptic a few times a day until it's healed.
☐	On airplane flights (or daily if your lymphedema is bad), wear a compression sleeve (on your arm) and a gauntlet (on your hand). See a lymphedema specialist to be measured properly, because wearing something too constricting might actually prove more harmful. Many women recommend the Juzo custom sleeve with silicon beads or the Juzo Dynamics or Juzo Dreamsleeve; Horst is also a preferred brand. • Lymphedema Products, (866) 445-9674, *www.LymphedemaProducts.com* • Compression Sale, (800) 504-7315, *www.CompressionSale.com* • Make Me Heal, (866) 363-4325, *www.MakeMeHeal.com*

	• Bright Life, *www.BrightLifeDirect.com* Therapists recommend **not** wearing a compression sleeve at night.
☐	Exercise regularly without straining your shoulder and arm.
☐	Avoid weight gain.
☐	Try lymphedema massage or lymphedema therapy.
☐	Some women find 'wrapping' successful; find a therapist who is trained. Wrapping (as opposed to compression sleeves) can be worn day and night.
☐	Some women have had success managing lymphedema using a range of complementary treatments from Thai yoga massage to aquatic therapy.
☐	Insurance plans may cover some of the costs of lymphedema massage and/or physical therapy. The cost of compression garments may also be covered.
☐	Consider wearing a lymphedema medical alert bracelet to remind medical personnel to avoid your arm in doing procedures. The bracelet should say: "No BP, no IV, no sticks—left arm" (rather than 'lymphedema'—because even many medical professionals won't know what

lymphedema is, and won't understand what they're not supposed to do. However, many women say that in a hospital situation, nobody checks your armband or bracelet anyway, so be sure it's written in big letters on your chart, keep a notice by your bedside with the same cautions, write it directly on the affected arm, and be sure you tell everyone involved in your care.)

- *www.shop.lymphnet.org/product.sc?productId=190*
- *www.tlcdirect.org/products/sku-8166__dept-40.html*
- *www.creativemedicalid.com/womens_medical_bracelets?b=1*

☐ Contact the Lymphedema Association of North America (LANA), *www.CLT-LANA.org,* or the National Lymphedema Network, *www.LymphNet.org,* for more information.

Checklist: Lymphedema Exercises

The following exercises may be helpful for your lymphedema, but consult a doctor or lymphedema specialist to be sure these are appropriate for your situation:

✓	Lymphedema Exercises
☐	Holding your arm above your head and heart, open and close your hand 25 times, 3-4 times a day.
☐	Standing with your face to the wall, place your hands on the wall just above your head and slowly 'walk' your fingers up the wall.
☐	Laying on your back, reach your hands high in front of your face, and hold, keeping your elbows straight. Lower the arm.
☐	Laying on your back, reach your hands high in front of your face, and then slowly lower them back behind your head, keeping your elbows straight.
☐	Sitting in a chair, place your palms together in front of you and press firmly.
☐	Sitting in a chair, 'shrug' your shoulders up towards your ears, hold, and then release.
☐	With your hands and feet on the ground in the all-fours position, lower your head to the ground,

	keeping your back straight. Then push yourself back up with your arms.
☐	With your hands and knees on the ground in the all-fours position, rock slowly back on your heels and lower your head down between your outstretched arms. Hold and return to the all-fours position.

When to Call Your Doctor

Contact your doctor if you experience any of the following:

- If your arm or underarm looks red, feels hot, or swells suddenly; you may have an infection or blood clot, or you may be developing cellulitis (which will require an antibiotic).

- If you have an (oral) fever of at least 100°F (38°C), unrelated to a cold or illness.

Fill-in: Lymphedema Log

Record situations which seem to trigger lymphedema, and any treatments you undergo for lymphedema, here.

Lymphedema Log			
Date	Situation	Treatment Date	Treatment
	Baseline arm measurements		

Date	Situation	Treatment Date	Treatment

The Clinical Trials Checklist

෴ ෴

Clinical trials are research studies (usually conducted by doctors or other medical personnel on human volunteers) designed to answer specific health questions. In terms of global health policy, clinical trials are an effective way to improve breast cancer care for the general population. Participating in a breast cancer clinical trial may allow you to receive innovative treatment that could become standard therapy, or let you gain access to experimental drugs when standard therapies are no longer effective.

Over the past 50 years, clinical trials have resulted in significant advances in many aspects of breast cancer care, but an inadequate number of volunteers is one of the major bottlenecks in drug development. Fewer than 5% of patients with cancer participate in clinical trials, due to lack of awareness.

In a clinical trial, you either receive the standard of care that is the most effective known treatment currently available (if you're in the control group) or a promising experimental treatment that might become standard care in the future.   There's no way to know whether any individual will benefit from the experimental treatment.

There are over 5000 clinical trials on breast cancer currently underway, on everything from quality of life studies to pain management.   If you're interested in considering participating in a clinical trial, ask your doctor and look at the following resources:

- National Cancer Institute:
  - *www.cancer.gov/clinicaltrials*

  - *www.cancer.gov/clinicaltrials/learningabout/treat ment-trial-guide*

  - (800) 4-CANCER—(800) 422-6237

  - *cancergovstaff@mail.nih.gov*

- *BreastCancerTrials.org*

- Center for Information and Study on Clinical Research Participation, *www.ciscrp.org*

The Post-Treatment Checklist

CB EO

You're done with treatment.

The labs have drawn your last blood, your chemotherapy port has been removed, and your oncologist has wished you well and said she'll see you once a year.

Your side-effects may persist (you may even acquire new ones) but you're basically done.

Tests such as blood tumor marker studies, blood tests of liver function, CT scans, bone scans, and chest X-rays are *not* part of standard follow-up care.

After five years of annual follow-ups, your oncologist probably won't need to see you at all anymore.

However, there are a few things you should be alert for:

Checklist: Post-Treatment

✓	Post-Treatment
☐	If you had a lumpectomy, ask your radiation oncologist if you should be monitored by MRI (see p 195).
☐	If you had breast-conserving surgery, you'll need a mammogram six months after radiation and then annually.
☐	If you had a mastectomy on one side, continue to have yearly mammograms on the other side.
☐	If you are taking Tamoxifen or Toremifene, and you are post-menopausal, you should have yearly pelvic exams because these drugs can increase your risk of uterine cancer. (Be sure to see your doctor immediately about any abnormal vaginal bleeding.)
☐	If you are taking an aromatase inhibitor, you may be at increased risk for thinning of the bones. Your doctor will want to monitor your bone health and may consider a bone density baseline test.
☐	If you recently discontinued use of aromatase inhibitors, you may still experience anxiety, mood swings, and/or depression.
☐	If you're triple-negative, you'll need oncology

	appointments every 3-6 months post-treatment (for 2 years), then every 6-12 months (for 3-4 years), and then once a year.
☐	If your doctor prescribes bisphosphonates (including Fosamax, Boniva, and Reclast) for bone health, ask if that's still recommended; the FDA just concluded that bisphosphonates may do more harm than good to women with bone density issues.
☐	If you've had silicone gel implants, ask your surgeon about getting regular MRIs to make sure the silicone isn't leaking; it doesn't always cause symptoms. Most women have their first MRI about a year after reconstruction, and then every two years after that. These MRIs may not be covered by insurance.
☐	If you've had a port implanted, be aware that it must be used (or flushed) every month, or it must be removed. Don't ignore this; leaving the port in without flushing it may lead to serious infection.
☐	If you have Taxol-induced neuropathy, your doctor may recommend Neurontin: Keep in mind that a common side-effect of Neurontin is memory loss. Some women also find vitamin E, calcium, and magnesium helpful for neuropathy.
☐	If you're interested in exploring the possibility of participating in a clinical trial, you can locate options

	at *www.Cancer.gov/clinicaltrials/search.*
☐	Many women find that their sex life changes post-surgery. Aside from all the emotional and psychological issues around losing your breast(s), and the fatigue issues that will plague you throughout treatment, chemotherapy will probably put you into (premature) menopause, and with less estrogen, your drive for sex will decrease. There are also practical issues, such as lack of lubrication. (Note that women who are on chemotherapy but also on certain antidepressants may have increased libido as a result.) One solution, for women whose husbands are disappointed in their lack of sexual interaction, is to try to increase intimacy other than through sexual intercourse: Spend more time snuggling together, or suggest a massage. Some couples also find seeing a therapist helpful.
☐	If you're suspected to be in a high risk group for genetic cancer (e.g., you're of Ashkenazic Jewish descent, or family members have tested positive for BRCA gene mutations, or family members have a history of breast, ovarian, or prostate cancer), ask your medical team about being tested for genetic mutations in the BRCA1 and BRCA2 genes. That will tell you whether your children are at risk for breast cancer, and will also tell you whether you have an increased risk for developing ovarian cancer and should consider a prophylactic oophorectomy

	(removal of the ovaries).
☐	When seeing a new doctor, or going to the hospital for any reason, make sure that everyone involved in your care knows not to use your affected arm for blood pressure, IVs, blood draws, or sticks. Be sure that this information is written *prominently* on your medical charts. And be sure you stay alert, so that you can yell if necessary :*) Some women recommend that, if you're going in for any procedure involving sedation, you write on your (affected) arm with a large red permanent marker "No IV, no BP, no sticks ON THIS ARM!" to prevent mistakes.

You would think that most cancer survivors would be ebullient and ecstatic when they reach the end of treatment. But ironically, many of us aren't.

After such an intense and depleting experience, it's hard, when your treatment finally ends, not to feel a sort of letdown, a disappointment, a sense of 'now what?'

Obviously finishing treatment is better than undergoing treatment. But many survivors are surprised by their feelings of dissatisfaction when suddenly treatment ends.

So be prepared.

Checklist: Getting On With Life

✓	Getting On With Life
☐	Do something to mark the end of your cancer journey: Throw a party, take a vacation, go on a meditation weekend.
☐	Mark the small milestones when you no longer have a treatment. For a year after my Herceptin treatments ended, every third Tuesday, when I would otherwise have been at Dana Farber in Boston, I went to a museum, out for lunch with a friend, or just gloried in sitting out in the sun reading a book.
☐	Consider throwing an annual 'cancer-versary' to celebrate the fact that you are now cancer-free. Invite friends over or out, or take a mini-vacation.
☐	Continue to eat healthfully and exercise regularly. Spend the time to develop a new nutritional and exercise plan, so that you don't slip back into bad habits.
☐	Similarly, don't slip back into your previous overscheduled and over-rushed lifestyle. You've probably learned something about your priorities as a result of your illness. Use this new knowledge to move forward and spend the time on relationships with family and friends.

☐	Give something back: Volunteer at a local cancer association, or become an online resource for friends and acquaintances dealing with cancer.
☐	Consider whether you want to in some little or large way thank the many people who helped you through the journey. You could: • Write thank you notes or emails to everyone. Don't forget the friends who cooked, schlepped, chauffeured, visited, lent you books and videos, and organized play dates for your children. • Take a few especially-helpful friends to lunch. • Bring fruit and goody baskets to the nurses in the chemotherapy ward and radiation room. • Send your oncologist and doctors a gift.
☐	Review your health insurance statements. Make sure you've been reimbursed for everything appropriately, and have submitted all necessary receipts.
☐	See if there are any remaining benefits on this year's health plan which you could utilize to alleviate symptoms or improve your overall physical condition. (I discovered that I was entitled to 30 free physical therapy sessions so I signed up for lymphedema massage and lymphedema aquatic therapy.)

☐	Consider going on one of the free or low-cost cancer survivor retreats (see p. 158) which for some can be a cathartic and helpful way to put this experience behind them, as well as a chance to really talk to others who've been on the same journey.
☐	Write in with your best tips for the cancer journey, and I'll try to share them in the next edition of this book. Email *info@BreastCancerChecklist.com*.

APPENDICES

Cʒ ꙮ

Contacts List

Cʒ ʒɔ

Here, keep all your non-medical contact information. (See the Medical Directory on p. 311 for medical contacts like doctors, nurses, lymphedema specialists, hospitals, pharmacies, etc.)

Contacts List	
Auto mechanic Name:	Phone:
Babysitter Name:	Phone:
Bank Name:	Phone:
Building superintendant Name:	Phone:
Cleaners Name:	Phone:
Handyman Name:	Phone:
Landlord Name:	Phone:
Neighbor Name:	Phone:

Taxicab Name:	Phone:
Teacher Name:	Phone:
Others:	
Name:	Phone:
Name:	Phone:
Name:	Phone:
Name:	Phone:
Name:	Phone:
Name:	Phone:
Name:	Phone:
Name:	Phone:
Name:	Phone:
Name:	Phone:

Menu Plans

❦ ❧

Here you can plan out menus ahead of time to make shopping and cooking easier for the whole family. See sample menu on p. 90.

Weekly Menu For _____		
	Lunch	**Dinner**
Sunday		
Monday		
Tuesday		
Wednesday		
Thursday		
Friday		
Saturday		

Sample Grocery List

೮ೞ ൈ

Shopping List		
Produce		**Spices**
Apples	Mushrooms-maitake	Anise
Apricots	Mushrooms-shiitake	Basil
Asparagus	Mushrooms-reishi	Bay leaves
Avocadoes	Onions	Black pepper
Banana	Oranges	Cardamom
Berries	Parsley	Cayenne pepper
Broccoli	Parsnips	Cilantro
Cabbage (green)	Peaches	Cinnamon
Cabbage (red)	Pears	Cloves
Carrots	Peppers	Coriander
Cauliflower	Pineapple	Cumin
Celery	Plums	Curry powder
Collard greens	Pomegranates	Dill
Cucumbers	Pumpkins	Fennel
Eggplants	Radishes	Ginger
Garlic	Raspberries	Nutmeg
Ginger root	Red onions	Oregano
Grapes	Scallions	Paprika
Kale	Squash	Parsley
Lemons	String beans	Red pepper
Lettuce	Sweet potatoes	Rosemary
Limes	Tomatoes	Tarragon
Melons	Watercress	Thyme
	Zucchini	Turmeric

Nuts/Seeds

Almonds
Chestnuts
Flax seed
Peanuts
Pecans
Pine nuts
Pumpkin seeds
Sesame seeds
Sunflower seeds
Walnuts

Beverages

Bottled water
Seltzer

Canned

Applesauce
Crushed tomatoes
Herring
Mackerel
Olives
Salmon
Sardines
Spaghetti sauce
Tomato paste
Tuna (canned)

Fresh fish

Household

Aluminum foil
Dish soap
Garbage bags
Kleenex
Laundry detergent
Napkins
Paper cups
Paper plates
Saran Wrap
Toilet paper
Toothpaste

Baking

Baking powder
Baking soda
Cocoa powder
Whole wheat flour
Whole wheat pastry
Yeast

Grains/Pasta

Barley
Bulgur wheat
Brown rice
Cereal-whole grain
Oatmeal (whole oats)
Whole couscous
Whole wheat bagels
Whole wheat bread
Whole wheat pasta

Beans

Aduki beans
Black beans
Chickpeas
Kidney beans
Lentils
Pinto beans
Split peas

Other

Coffee
Green tea
Humus
Olive oil
Salt
Sesame oil
Vinegar
Whole-wheat crackers

Seaweed

Arame
Dulse
Hijiki
Kelp
Kombu
Nori
Wakame

Other items
needed this week:

Items You've Borrowed

CB EO

Here, keep track of books, DVDs, and other items you've borrowed and need to return:

Items Borrowed			
Date	From	Item	Returned?

Date	From	Item	Returned?

Gifts and Assistance

C3 80

Keep track of who's helped you and how:

Gifts and Assistance		
Date	Name	Gift / Helped Out How

Date	Name	Gift / Helped Out How

Health Insurance Plan Summary

CR ₿O

Here keep just the highlights of your health insurance plan, so that you can easily find details when necessary:

Health Insurance Plan Summary	
Insurance company	
Plan name	
Policy number	
Address	
Telephone	
Fax	
E-mail	
Second opinion included?	

Annual deductible	
Co-pays	Primary care physician: _____ Specialist: _____ Emergency room: _____
Covered hospital costs	
Days of hospital coverage	
Cost of prescribed drugs	
Physical therapy visits per year	
Prostheses coverage	Breast forms:_____ Wig:_____ Bra:_____

Insurance Company Interactions

❧ ☙

Here, maintain a detailed list of all interactions with your insurance company. Keep an accompanying folder to hold all the receipts, invoices, statements, and referral letters. Be sure to get the insurance authorization number for any treatment for which you might later need proof of approval. For each interaction by telephone, record:

Insurance Company Interactions		
Date & Time	Name & Title	Summary, including Authorization Number

Date & Time	Name & Title	Summary, including Authorization Number

Date & Time	Name & Title	Summary, including Authorization Number

Date & Time	Name & Title	Summary, including Authorization Number

Insurance Receipts

෪ ෫

Keep a record of all your health-related expenses here, so that you have everything you need for insurance reimbursement or tax refunds.

Insurance Receipts				
Date	Item	$	Date Insurance Paid	Amount Insurance Paid

306 Insurance Receipts

Date	Item	$	Date Insurance Paid	Amount Insurance Paid

Transportation Records

⍣ ⍥

Keep track of mileage and/or expenses associated with each trip to doctors, hospitals, diagnostic tests, physical therapy appointments, pharmacies, etc., all of which might be able to be written off your taxes.

Transportation Records			
Date	Destination	Purpose	Expense / Mileage

Date	Destination	Purpose	Expense / Mileage

Pharmacy Purchases

ଓ ଯୋ

Keep track of pharmacy-related expenses, that is, money spent for medicines and other non-drug items like bandages that you purchased for your treatment, as these might be able to be written off your taxes.

Date	Prescription	Prescribed By	Expense

Pharmacy Purchases

310 Pharmacy Purchases

Date	Prescription	Prescribed By	Expense

Medical Directory

Cʒ ꙮ

Include listings for all your doctors, nurses, lymphedema therapists, etc.—everyone involved in your care, so that you can locate their information quickly when you need it.

Medical Directory	
Name	
Name of practice	
Address	
Specialty	
Phone/fax	
E-mail address	
Name	
Name of practice	
Address	

Specialty	
Phone/fax	
E-mail address	
Name	
Name of practice	
Address	
Specialty	
Phone/fax	
E-mail address	
Name	
Name of practice	
Address	
Specialty	
Phone/fax	
E-mail address	
Name	

Name of practice	
Address	
Specialty	
Phone/fax	
E-mail address	
Name	
Name of practice	
Address	
Specialty	
Phone/fax	
E-mail address	
Name	
Name of practice	
Address	
Specialty	
Phone/fax	

E-mail address	
Name	
Name of practice	
Address	
Specialty	
Phone/fax	
E-mail address	
Name	
Name of practice	
Address	
Specialty	
Phone/fax	
E-mail address	

Treatment Summary

ℭ℥ ℬ℧

Here, track important dates of your treatment, so that you can recall them at a glance. In addition to this chart, you should file the following:

- *A copy of your biopsy pathology report*

- *A copy of your surgery pathology report*

- *A copy of the hospital discharge summary*

- *A copy of the chemotherapy summary*

- *A copy of the radiation summary*

Find details of:

- *Surgeries on p. 321*

- *Diagnostic tests on p. 325*

- *Medications on p. 339*

- *Doctor appointments on p. 333*

Treatment Summary		
Date of birth		
Age at first diagnosis		
Family history of cancer		
How cancer first discovered (lump? mammogram?), and date		
Biopsy date		
	Left side	Right side
Type of cancer (from biopsy pathology report)		
Estrogen / progesterone receptor positive / negative (from biopsy pathology		

report)		
HER2/neu-positive (from biopsy pathology report)		
Stage of cancer (from biopsy pathology report)		
Tumor grade (from biopsy pathology report)		
Surgery date		
	Left side	Right side
Number of cancerous lymph nodes discovered		
Number of lymph nodes removed in total		
Type of cancer (from post-surgery pathology report)		
Estrogen / progesterone		

receptor positive / negative (from post-surgery pathology report)		
HER2/neu-positive (from post-surgery pathology report)		
Stage of cancer (from post-surgery pathology report)		
Tumor grade (from post-surgery pathology report)		
Infusion port surgery date		
Start date of chemotherapy		
Chemotherapy regimen—drugs, amounts		
Start date of radiation		
Start date of		

Herceptin, and dose	
Start date of Tamoxifen / aromatase inhibitor, and dose	
Clinical trial participation	
Additional notes	

Surgery Record

CG ᙎ

Include listings for all surgery performed, including lumpectomy, mastectomy, reconstruction, infusion port, etc.

Surgery Record	
Date	
Type of surgery	
Name of surgeon	
Results / Be alert for	
Follow-up plan	

Date	
Type of surgery	
Name of surgeon	
Results / Be alert for	
Follow-up plan	
Date	
Type of surgery	
Name of surgeon	
Results / Be alert for	

Follow-up plan	
Date	
Type of surgery	
Name of surgeon	
Results / Be alert for	
Follow-up plan	

Diagnostic Tests Record

❧ ☙

Include listings for all diagnostic tests, including X-rays, CT scans, ultrasounds, echocardiograms, blood tests, MRIs, mammograms, etc. so that you can easily locate this information when you need it.

Diagnostic Tests	
Type of test	
Date	
Testing facility	
Name of doctor or professional	
Telephone	
E-mail	
Date results available	

How to obtain results	
How to follow-up?	
Type of test	
Date	
Testing facility	
Name of doctor or professional	
Telephone	
E-mail	
Date results available	
How to obtain results	
How to follow-up?	
Type of test	

Date	
Testing facility	
Name of doctor or professional	
Telephone	
E-mail	
Date results available	
How to obtain results	
How to follow-up?	
Type of test	
Date	
Testing facility	
Name of doctor or professional	
Telephone	

E-mail	
Date results available	
How to obtain results	
How to follow-up?	
Type of test	
Date	
Testing facility	
Name of doctor or professional	
Telephone	
E-mail	
Date results available	
How to obtain results	

How to follow-up?	
Type of test	
Date	
Testing facility	
Name of doctor or professional	
Telephone	
E-mail	
Date results available	
How to obtain results	
How to follow-up?	
Type of test	
Date	
Testing facility	

Name of doctor or professional	
Telephone	
E-mail	
Date results available	
How to obtain results	
How to follow-up?	

Bone Density Records

❦ ❧

Record your bone density readings, starting with a baseline (before treatment) reading, to track osteoporosis.

Bone Density Records	
Date	**Reading**
	Baseline bone density reading:

Date	Reading

Doctor Appointments

CB EO

Record all the details of your medical appointments.

Doctor Appointments	
Date	
Doctor's name	
Symptoms, problems, side-effects to discuss	
Notes from visit	
Date	
Doctor's name	
Symptoms, problems, side-	

effects to discuss	
Notes from visit	
Date	
Doctor's name	
Symptoms, problems, side-effects to discuss	
Notes from visit	
Date	
Doctor's name	
Symptoms, problems, side-effects to discuss	

Notes from visit	
Date	
Doctor's name	
Symptoms, problems, side-effects to discuss	
Notes from visit	
Date	
Doctor's name	
Symptoms, problems, side-effects to discuss	

Notes from visit	
Date	
Doctor's name	
Symptoms, problems, side-effects to discuss	
Notes from visit	
Date	
Doctor's name	
Symptoms, problems, side-effects to discuss	

Notes from visit	
Date	
Doctor's name	
Symptoms, problems, side-effects to discuss	
Notes from visit	
Date	
Doctor's name	
Symptoms, problems, side-effects to discuss	

Notes from visit	
Date	
Doctor's name	
Symptoms, problems, side-effects to discuss	
Notes from visit	

Medications

CƷ ꙮ

Record all the details of the medicines you are taking, including over-the-counter medicines (e.g. aspirin), herbs, and prescribed-medicine.

Medicines		
Name of Medication	Side-Effects to Monitor	When to Take (with/without food, time of day)

Name of Medication	Side-Effects to Monitor	When to Take (with/without food, time of day)

Follow-Up Schedule

ℭℬ ℬↄ

Here you can record your follow-up schedule of future doctor appointments, periodic tests, and other events. See The Post-Treatment Checklist on p. 280 for more details on follow-up guidelines.

Follow-Up Schedule	
Date to schedule	**Doctor: (for what procedure)**
1st Year	
	Surgeon (6-month follow-up)
	Oncologist (annual appointment; or every 3-6 months for triple-negative women)
	Annual pelvic exam (if on Tamoxifen)
	Annual mammogram (if you had breast-conserving surgery, unilateral mastectomy or lumpectomy)

	MRI scan (if you have silicone gel implants)
	Bone density scan (if you're taking aromatase inhibitors or Tamoxifen)

2nd Year	
	Oncologist (annual appointment; or every 3-6 months for triple-negative women)
	Annual pelvic exam (if on Tamoxifen)
	Annual mammogram (if you had breast-conserving surgery, unilateral mastectomy, or lumpectomy)
	Bone density scan (if you're taking aromatase inhibitors or Tamoxifen)

3rd Year	
	Oncologist (annual appointment; or every 6-12 months for triple-negative women)
	Annual pelvic exam (if on Tamoxifen)
	Annual mammogram (if you had breast-conserving surgery, unilateral mastectomy, or lumpectomy)
	MRI scan (if you have silicone gel implants)
	Bone density scan (if you're taking aromatase inhibitors or Tamoxifen)
4th Year	
	Oncologist (annual appointment; or every 6-12 months for triple-negative women)

	Annual pelvic exam (if on Tamoxifen)
	Annual mammogram (if you had breast-conserving surgery, unilateral mastectomy, or lumpectomy)
	Bone density scan (if you're taking aromatase inhibitors or Tamoxifen)

5th Year

	Oncologist (annual appointment; or every 6-12 months for triple-negative women)
	Annual pelvic exam (if on Tamoxifen)
	Annual mammogram (if you had breast-conserving surgery, unilateral mastectomy, or lumpectomy)
	MRI scan (if you have silicone gel implants)
	Bone density scan (if you're taking

	aromatase inhibitors or Tamoxifen)

Resources

CB BO

Here are additional helpful resources:

- The American Cancer Society, *Cancer.org*

- National Cancer Institute:
  - *www.Cancer.gov*
  - *(800) 4-CANCER—(800) 422-6237*
  - *cancergovstaff@mail.nih.gov*

- Susan G. Komen for the Cure, *www.komen.org*

- Dr. Susan Love Research Foundation, *dslrf.org*

- *breastcancer.org*

- Dana-Farber Cancer Institute, *www.dana-farber.org*

- M. D. Anderson Cancer Center, *www.mdanderson.org*

- The Mayo Clinic, *www.mayoclinic.com*

- Memorial Sloan-Kettering Cancer Center, *www.mskcc.org*

- Oncolink, *www.Oncolink.org*. Managed by the University of Pennsylvania

- *ParentingwithCancer.com* is a website with helpful articles on parenting through cancer treatment.

- You can fill out your family health history with the government's free online tool at *FamilyHistory.hhs.gov.*

- You can check the current recommendations for treating your type of breast cancer at *www.nccn.org*, The National Comprehensive Cancer Network.

- Women concerned about cancer treatments affecting their fertility should be in touch with Fertile Hope, *FertileHope.org*, (888) 994-2353, or the Oncofertility Consortium (*Oncofertility.northwestern.edu*) hotline, (866) 708-3378. *MyOncoFertility.org* is another resource for patients provided by the Oncofertility Consortium.

- If your children would benefit from a support group geared to kids whose parents have cancer, *www.ChildrensTreeHouseFdn.org/support.html* offers listings.

- Breast Cancer Social Media Tweet Chat, Monday nights at 9pm ET, on Twitter (follow *@BCSMComm, bcsm.info*)

- There are many online sites that can assist communities in organizing play dates, carpools, and food; they also include message boards where friends can post greetings. These include:

- o   *www.CaringBridge.org*
- o   *www.LotsaHelpingHands.com*
- o   *www.TakeThemAMeal.com*
- o   *www.MealTrain.com*

- The Neuropathy Association, (212) 692-0662, *www.Neuropathy.org*

- The Lymphedema Association of North America (LANA), *www.CLT-LANA.org,* and the National Lymphedema Network *www.LymphNet.org*

- Locate clinical trial possibilities at:

  - o   *www.Cancer.gov/clinicaltrials*
  - o   *www.Cancer.gov/clinicaltrials/search*
  - o   *www.Cancer.gov/clinicaltrials/learningabout/treatment-trial-guide*
  - o   *BreastCancerTrials.org*

- The Living Beyond Breast Cancer Survivors' Helpline at (888) 753-5222

- The Triple-Negative Helpline, (877) 880-8622

- Find prosthesis info at *Breastfree.org*.

- Complementary cancer care information can be found at:

  o National Cancer Institute Office of Complementary and Alternative Medicine, *cam.cancer.gov/cam/health_patients.html*

  o Memorial Sloan Kettering Cancer Center, *www.mskcc.org/cancer-care/integrative-medicine*

  o University of Texas M.D. Anderson Cancer Center Complementary/Integrative Medicine Educational Resources, *www.mdanderson.org/CIMER*

Index

೫ ೩

About the Author

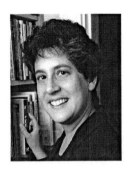

Fern Reiss is an honors graduate of Harvard University. She is the author of *The Publishing Game: Publish a Book in 30 Days, The Publishing Game: Find an Agent in 30 Days, The Publishing Game: Bestseller in 30 Days, The Publishing Game: Internet Publicity in 30 Days, The Publishing Game: Blog Tours in 30 Days, Terrorism and Kids: Comforting Your Child,* and *The Infertility Diet: Get Pregnant and Prevent Miscarriage,* all published by PublishingGame.com/PBJ Press.

Fern helps authors and CEOs publish and promote books (*PublishingGame.com*) and helps businesses and organizations get better media attention (*Expertizing.com*.) She is on the board of directors of both the Harvard Alumni Association and Harvard Entrepreneurial Startups, and is a member of the American Society of Journalists and Authors. She is a popular conference speaker on publishing, publicity, and entrepreneurship. She lives with her husband and three children in Boston.

The Breast Cancer Checklist is available at *BreastCancerChecklist.com*, online, and at local bookstores and libraries everywhere.

If you'd like to order a large quantity of books for a doctor's office, hospital, or organization, please contact us directly:

PublishingGame.com
Peanut Butter and Jelly Press, LLC
PO Box 590239, Newton, MA 02459-0002
orders@PublishingGame.com
(617) 630-0945

CPSIA information can be obtained at www.ICGtesting.com
Printed in the USA
LVOW101013200213

320914LV00001B/35/P

9 781893 290204